Healthy Medicine

The Philosophy and Principles of Natural Medicine

By

Dr Bernard Brom

Healthy Medicine

Published by:
Kima Global Publishers
50, Clovelly Road
Clovelly
7975
South Africa

© 2016 Dr. Bernard Brom

ISBN: 978-1-920535-92-6
eISBN 978-1-920535-93-3

Publisher's web site: www.kimabook.com
Author's web site: www.creatinghealth.co.za

Cover photograph © Dave Cole

Dedication

I would like to dedicate this book to all the patients who came to see me over the many years I practised my art of medicine. I am sure it was not easy for all of them: there were times I was radical, and then times of confusion as I tried to define a new path for myself in a medicine that had crystalised itself into what I regarded as rigid, narrow-minded and stuck in a dogmatic interpretation of illness that did not fit mine.

My patients encouraged me in the process. They too were dissatisfied with doctors who were only interested in the disease, who gave them drugs that had serious side-effects and refused to listen to their deeper questioning.

Together we forged a new path, and this book is the result.

Thanks also to my dear wife, Jeanne, who read through the many versions, correcting my sometimes poor handling of English grammar, and constantly encouraging me to complete this work. I am deeply grateful.

Table of Contents

Foreword

After Descartes, science changed the world view of reality and Western medicine followed to end up focusing on the human body and ignoring the human person within complex relationships. Since Einstein and the birth of quantum physics science has changed but medicine is still dominated by the modernity mind of Descartes.

In the last 80 years many thought leaders in medicine have tried to take medicine out of this capture by a limited view of reality by modern science. Paul Tournier, Michael Balint, Ian McWhinney and many others have shown how people are better healed when we go beyond narrow measurable science and give attention to relationships and subjectivity. However their influence has not gone very far beyond the development of Family Medicine within the dominant medical system still operating today.

In Healthy Medicine Bernard Brom adds his voice to the many others before him to bring the practice of medicine back from working with bodies to being fit for complex persons in community and environment. He paints a picture of why medicine is not following the new science and the wisdom from experience over thousands of years. The book describes his search for the Principles and Philosophy for the kind of medicine that is fit for wellness and healing. It is a graphic description of a personal, inward and outward journey to bring the reader to the point of Bernard's finding of what medicine should be like. The views expressed are often denigrated and viciously opposed by the mainline system in medicine today but it seems that this journey is taking shape with many more across the world joining the practice of Integrative or Natural Medicine.

This book offers readers much in understanding the inner journey Bernard had to take to come to his comprehensive understanding of where we have gone wrong and where we need to reroute for the future of medicine that will be fit for purpose. We cannot move out of the present mode of function dominating medicine without the inner journey that changes the healer. In the outer journey Bernard also discovered many approaches and therapies that need to be considered. It is not a rejection of science but rather scientism that ignores all that it cannot measure. So the promoted future mode of function is one in which the constricted vision of science is not ignored but where the wisdom from experience is given an equal footing where we remain humble in the face of uncertainty and the Great Mystery beyond our measurement instruments. Bernard's journey brought him a long way from moving away from focusing on symptoms and disease to deal with underlying causes and re-harmonising toward wellness.

Samuel Fehrsen, former professor of Family Practice Medunsa and Consultant in Health Professions Education and Primary Health Care.

Introduction

It has been a long day and the sun has just begun to set, casting a pink shadow on the mountains. Up in the valley there are no sunsets, only the shadows reflecting the changing patterns of light. It seems that sometimes we never see directly but must rely on shadows, reflections, and signs and other manifestations of that which is always hidden from our view.

I have learnt with the passage of time that the world I see, smell, hear and touch is but a fleeting glimpse of some much deeper truth. I now know that this truth dances away as I stretch to touch it but that it yields to me some of its perfume if I stop trying so hard to understand.

The whole of my professional life has been about seeking a deeper truth. It seems that something very deep inside me knows that what I know is just a very small part of the whole. In that journey of seeking a deeper truth I have discovered certain principles and laws which govern the flow of life, slowly developing a philosophy around these principles and laws bringing it all into a cohesive and understandable whole. What I practice is called Integrative Medicine but in the larger context it is part of 'natural medicine'.

A great deal has been written about natural medicine, in books, in articles, seminars, radio talk shows etc., but in general all this information has to do with techniques, remedies, tests and methods of application. Every year new techniques and new disciplines appear in the health care arena, which are claimed to be more effective than others. Old remedies are re-discovered, ancient scriptures translated and new meaning attached to traditional methods.

In the plethora of old and new ideas it is the principles and philosophy common to all which are often forgotten.

There is a good reason for this. Many health practitioners themselves get caught up in the same Western style materialistic and reductionistic paradigm in which techniques and treating disease is the most important consideration. Many practitioners attend weekend courses and then start practising.

Weekend courses do not teach philosophy and principles, but techniques, which can give quick results. Patients themselves tend to think that the only difference between natural medicine and conventional medicine is that in the former one uses natural medicines and in the latter one uses drugs to treat the disease. Even many practitioners of natural medicine are unaware of the enormous difference that exists between these two disciplines. The difference is more than skin deep. There is a profound and very significant difference between traditional systems of healing, natural medical approaches and the way modern medicine interprets health and disease.

In this book we will be trying to capture the heart of this difference. This book is not about techniques or remedies, but much more about the principles, which underpin these techniques.

It would seem that any understanding of techniques and methods of treatment is only possible if the principles underlining these methods are understood. It is also possible that once this understanding is in place, then one may begin to see a common thread, which runs through all these techniques.

This in fact was my own personal experience. During my first few years in the practice of natural medicine I became more and more excited with the wonderful world of exciting new methods and treatment options that became available to me. My library of books soon filled, my shelves became overstocked with all kinds of natural medicines and in each room was a different machine to treat ill health including light therapy, magnetic therapy and various electromagnetic applications.

Soon however I became a little confused about which method was best and which remedy to use. What astonished me was the fact that all methods and systems seem to give results. It seemed that some techniques were better than other techniques for certain clearly defined conditions but nevertheless there were always numerous options and a great deal of overlap.

At this point of my learning curve I decided that there must be some common principles involved. It did not seem possible that all these methods were using different underlying tenets. If I could find the common principles then perhaps this would help me in deciding what was best for each patient.

I once asked a Professor of Medicine what he regarded as most important in the teaching of medical students. The bottom line, he said, was 'science' and more science. I don't agree with this statement. My own experience has led me to believe that experience accumulated over years together with that of thousands of other doctors doing similar work is as important as the science which supports this experience.

Will more science resolve the world problems? What about 'experience'?

It is often over tea discussing one's experience with colleagues that new ideas are born. My 35 years of experience with the low energy laser started at a seminar learning about acupuncture. The colleague sitting next to me kept suggesting that needles were not the only way to stimulate acupuncture points. He was a homeopath and during the tea break invited me to his rooms to watch him work.

I spent three days watching in amazement how he used the laser instead of needles to stimulate acupuncture points but he also used the laser in a range of other conditions with extraordinary results. There were no text books easily available at that time; nevertheless just watching and being open minded to this new tool was enough for me to order my first low-energy laser.

It took me less than one month to become convinced of its usefulness and not more than 6 months to develop an expertise in its use. By the time I received the first textbook in the use of low energy laser therapy I was surprised at how much I had learnt through experience and indeed how much I could have taught the author about new ways of using the laser. So much for experience. Waiting for the science to catch up with my experience could probably have taken many years indeed and held back my contribution to patients' wellness.

It is not clear whether the ancients sitting around the fire or staring out over the plains watching the movement of buffalo or elephants indulged in philosophical discussion but certainly they studied the movement of the winds, the flow of the seasons, the growth and then disappearance of the moon, the awesomeness of a woman giving birth, the mystery of a spider web and the house building of bees and termites. In order to survive they needed to know these things and they could feel in their own bodies the flow of the day and the cycle of change.

There was order here in this streaming of time and the 'law of nature' needed to be respected.

One of my acupuncture teachers was taught by his father starting when he was only about 9 years of age. When he returned home from school he would spend some time with his father carrying the tray of needles and watching his father work. There was no conventional teaching, as we understand it in the west, just watching. This went on for many years until one day his father handed him a needle and told him to insert the needle into a particular acupuncture point. This is the way of traditional systems of healing i.e. apprenticing with a known master and often travelling around to find other masters who could take one to another level.

When I was in China, I went out of my way to meet some of the old master acupuncturists (a dying breed) and was astonished to discover how differently each one practiced.

There were of course many similarities but I could understand why it was necessary to travel around and discover each person's unique approach to different conditions. Today Traditional Chinese Medicine has been standardised so that in all the very numerous Schools of TCM the students are all taught the same curriculum. Nevertheless there is an attempt to maintain a creative edge by allowing individual experimentation based on the practitioner's experience taking place within the TCM colleges.

While I am clearly not suggesting that experience alone is enough to drive progress in medicine, it does need to move hand in hand with experiment and the science of medicine. I am concerned that today there are serious attempts to restrict that creative edge unless it fits within the known and conventional practice of medicine. While doctors today may be expert technicians and can use very powerful drugs to control symptoms, the fact is that in general people's health is not improving. There is more and more chronic disease and very little understanding in turning ill health back to perfect health. More and more individuals rely on drugs just to get them through the day.

We have moved from experience guiding our life to expecting science to resolve all our problems.

So in the beginning was contemplation, musing, debates, fireside chats, inspiration and meaningful experiences in nature etc. through which one derives meaning, significance, essence and purpose and reaches out towards making all this work in healing the patient.

Along this journey the observant practitioner begins to see common principles and slowly develops the background philosophy to support those principles. The philosophy and principles underlying the practice of natural methods of healing become the guiding teaching of today's natural approaches to ill health.

There is a tendency by many academics to think that medical students should not have to bother with philosophy and principle of healing but just get on with the job of treating disease. It seems that Professors of Medicine believe that students must keep their feet on the ground and deal with the real issues of suffering mankind.

Medical students today are taught by medical specialists who generally are less interested in the person and more interested in the disease. The concept of biopsychosocial medicine has arisen within the corridors of family practice and not within those of specialist medicine. Family practitioners are trying to return the patient back to the centre of medicine rather than the focus on the disease.

It may surprise many of us to discover that in ancient times there were already great schools of learning, famous teachers, naturalist philosophers, scholars, historians. For example Confucius, the most famous Chinese philosopher was born in 552 BCE and his teaching focused on human behaviour, moral issues and how to live a virtuous life.

The first book about acupuncture, the Nei Jing was written during the Warring States period (403-221 BCE) and focused on major theoretical concepts and theories. Perhaps being closer to nature than we are today and having to rely on weather, the flow of the seasons, watching the movement of the sun and moon, the power of floods and storms, the movement of change and the recognition of an underlying order brought the wise men and women of the time to the understanding that there were laws of nature that one needed to respect. The study of these laws and the way of nature helped these great thinkers to formulate principles of health and good living.

Nature was and is and will continue to be a great teacher.

The history and development of healing and medicine emerged out of such a process. From very simple beginnings and a close observation of nature and the laws which pertained to it, human beings developed an understanding of the way towards healing and health. A system of healing only developed when deeper questions were asked and a philosophy of the healing process developed, leading to the principles related to that particular philosophical school of thought.

The powerful influence of modern scientific thinking has contributed enormously to our understanding of health and ill health. Nevertheless when scientific thinking dominates over the experience of practitioners then it can become dogmatic and narrow minded. This is called 'scientism' rather than science. Scientists are not isolated from their own feelings, inspiration and intuition and these subjective influences are always present as they do their science of measurement. Just acknowledging this would go a long way to bringing the 'science' of experience back into the fold of medicine.

My personal story

As we progress through the chapters we will be working through my own personal journey from a very ordinary and Western trained medical doctor to becoming an holistic practitioner using natural medicines to treat ill health. The journey I took when I gave up conventional medicine in 1971 had no special route in the beginning. I was unhappy and dissatisfied with life and blamed it on the fact that I had chosen the wrong profession.

Leaving medicine and travelling around the world as an artist did not immediately resolve my unhappiness. After a few months the same cycles of depression returned. Despite the beauty and tranquillity of the places we were visiting and despite the fact that there was no immediate pressure on me to find work as we had saved up sufficient funds and there was no difficulty as a doctor to find part time work, my general unhappiness continued.

At first I blamed my companion for my unhappiness, the place we were living in, my inability to find self-expression in artwork, the local inhabitants who were unfriendly and didn't understand me. There was no end of causes for the unhappiness and then, one day, I had the most astonishing revelation. We were living in one of Gods special gifts to mankind; a beautiful island with the most friendly islanders and coral reefs that stretched in all directions.

There were no excuses now and no one to blame as I stared out to sea. The emerald green of the water seemed to reflect my image back to me and I wondered for the first time if the problem of my own unhappiness lay within rather than out there. Could I be the problem? It was the first time that it occurred to me that it wasn't people or places that were responsible for my unhappiness but rather my philosophical outlook on life, which influenced my attitude towards people and places.

Once I began to change my expectation and my attitude towards places and people, I discovered that my depressive moods became fewer and there was a general feeling of well being and inner peace that had not been there before. I realised that I was in control of my inner space and I began to organise that inner space differently.

Secondly, in my travels around the world I was astonished to discover and see for myself so many different ways of treating people. In Europe all the young people I met were talking about organic food, using herbs, bottled water, home baked bread, homeopathic medicines, yoga and meditation.

In America I came across New Age energy machines, which used colour, light, laser and electrical pulsation to treat disease. In India I learned the power of the mind over matter and in China the use of needles to maintain health and treat disease.

Suddenly, a whole new way of seeing health and disease opened up before me. It was like discovering a new restaurant with food you had never tasted before in your own neighbourhood. I had found a direction and focus in my life.

In retrospect I realise now that from that moment I began to move in two quite different directions. There was an outward movement towards discovering more methods and techniques for treating disease and an inward movement towards discovering more about myself and the nature of my inner space. These two movements have continued without interruption since that time, feeding each other and often being the catalyst for further growth and understanding.

As I learnt more and more techniques there was always the nagging question of 'What is the common principle involved here?' I could not believe that all these systems of healing and techniques of treatment did not have something in common. I moved from one to the other searching for meaning in each and recognising that the only common factors were the practitioner and the patient.

I believe that something happens between the practitioner and the patient that is of a very special nature and may have an enormous influence on the outcome of the treatment process. I will deal with this in later chapters.

The other movement my journey took was an internal one. It started off very simply in trying to discover why I was unhappy.

In searching for the underlying cause, and for meaning in life, I slowly began to formulate certain principles regarding the nature of thought, which helped me to understand and gain clarification later of healing principles. It seemed to me that my inner life and principles, which applied to that inner life was somehow also reflected in my outer life and the circumstances and synchronicity of each moment.

This book is not about my inner journey, yet it is not possible to ignore this journey in my many discussions of health and disease. The inner and outer space seem almost to breathe in and out of each other, feeding and nourishing, moving and motivating so that I have great difficulty in keeping them apart.

I may appear at times to dwell too long on what appears to be philosophical issues. Be careful about ignoring these issues. They help one to enter the inner space as it were, to step back and to 'look out' onto the wider world with a clearer vision. There is a real need today for this to take place. Too many people are seeking only technique without clarity of the process. By seeking principle and coming constantly back to philosophy and the principles that emerge we can slowly bring together all these different techniques and come to a proper and good integration of all these different systems for the benefit of the ill person.

As we move from chapter to chapter the principles of health and disease will slowly emerge but we first need to discover who this human being is that became ill and then we need to find out how does this happen.

Along this journey we also need to try to keep in touch with the great mystery and remember that there is more we don't know than what we know. Hopefully this truth will prevent us from becoming dogmatic and narrow-minded. What we don't know may never be knowable and yet will constantly keep driving us to ask questions and seek deeper truths. If this book leaves you with more questions than answers then it will have served part of its purpose.

Chapter 1

I am angry. Reading how big multinational companies have placed profit above public safety and often in collusion with politicians, stirs up a deep anger towards people that are more concerned about the bottom line of profit making than human health. The story of how genetically modified foods (GMF) have been introduced into the public food supply is an example of the worst kind. The selling of cigarettes to innocent people, especially children, with the knowledge we have today is another.

With GMF we have a deliberate attempt from the beginning to confuse and to bypass the normal safety channels. Information was suppressed and deliberately contorted and attempts were made to present part of the story only, giving an impression that studies showed that GMF were safe to use when very clearly this was not exactly what all studies had showed. In fact there is good evidence that the opposite is true. Many substantial studies showed that GMF could be dangerous to our health, yet every effort was made to get these products into the market place as fast as possible before too much evidence as to their safety was available.

It is not difficult to understand that if one introduces a novel man made food product into the market that the long term consequences could be seriously problematic. Cancer takes 10 to 20 years to develop and this also applies to many of the chronic diseases we see today. Research of only a few months in animals cannot possible give such long term prediction of harm or harmlessness and even a few studies showing harm should raise alarm bells. It is really not good enough that some short term studies showing safety should satisfy professionals in the face of the real possibility that genetic modification is touching the very heart of the cell structure.

GM crops have not been proven unconditionally safe and there is sufficient evidence to make many good scientists wary of this process. With this huge question mark around GM products, allowing them to be used freely by human beings and especially children is experimental. It is the kind of science that should not be allowed. Why would companies selling GM derived foods not want that information available clearly on the package.

Rats fed GM potatoes have shown serious defects. The rats suffered damaged immune systems; the thymus and spleen showed evidence of damage and some of the rats had smaller, less developed brains, livers and testicles. There were other defects that were interesting and of some concern. Some of the GM potatoes were nutritionally different to their non-GM parent lines even though they were grown in identical conditions.

Man's mind it seems, is not nature's mind and the result of genetic manipulation was exactly that... manipulation without seeing the bigger picture. Biological Science is still too limited. We know far too little about the way nature works to interfere with the very source of life...the genetic map and codes.

This problem of GMF should be a clear warning about interfering with nature and so the discussion of what is natural has become more relevant in recent times as chemists, big business and governments become more involved in controlling and defining how food, nutritional supplements and herbs should be regulated.

What is Natural Medicine?

This book is about natural medicine and the way that medical doctors are 'integrating' these principles into their practice of medicine. In this chapter we will confine our attention to some broad issues and in particular try and define what the word 'natural' actually means.

Natural medicine is a system of medicine that focuses on prevention of illness and the use of non-toxic, natural therapies in the treatment and management of ill health.

It seems that most professionals like to steer away from defining the word 'natural' so that a discussion can no longer be left to chance. The word may appear on many diverse products and be used to include a multitude of events, objects and even emotions.

Natural[1]:

- Of or arising from nature
- Produced or existing in nature; not artificial

1   Collins dictionary

- As found in nature: unaltered by man

A herbal medicine may be natural, but is its active ingredient when separated by chemists still natural? Is an alcoholic tincture of the herb natural and can the herb be separated into its constituent parts and then put together again in order to control the chemical constituents still be regarded as natural?

There are good reasons for doing all this to natural substances. It is well known that the chemical constituents of plants will vary during the year and according to the weather conditions. Doctors need to be sure that what they give their patients has sufficient active ingredients to do the job required. As we process the herb more and more, trying to remove the most active parts of the herb, it very often begins to look more like a drug than a natural herbal substance.

The herb is extremely complex while the drug is a pretty simple chemical structure by comparison. While it may make sense that the so called 'active' ingredient part of the plant is all that is required, this may nevertheless be an assumption based on our limited understanding of plants and herbs and how these are processed in the body.

Vitamins and minerals are generally thought of as single isolated substances but that is not how they appear within the plant structure. Water for example is hydrogen and oxygen but they do not exactly appear as single isolated elements within water but rather blend into each other in a unique way. Vitamins and minerals are also blended into the structure of the plant.

Most vitamins found in supplements are synthesised from petroleum derivatives or hydrogenated sugars. So even though they are called natural and regarded as identical to the natural vitamins found in foods there are good reasons to question these assumptions.

How should one consider processed foods such as corn flakes made from natural ingredients, fortified brown health bread, tinned food, and alcoholic beverages? These foods do not obviously grow out of the ground and yet will often carry the label 'natural' on them. Fruit juices are often heated to sterilise the contents at temperatures, which destroy its natural vitamins and enzymes. They carry labels such as 'natural', free of preservatives and colourants, but are they natural…as found in nature: unaltered by man?

Food is heated in microwave ovens, which may change its organic structure. These changes may be too subtle to detect at present. The destructive effects of X-rays on living systems were only noted many years after their discovery. This kind of radiation is now used to destroy cancer cells.

So there are huge questions around the definition of 'natural' and what should be regarded as a genuine natural substance. Does it really make a difference if it is synthetically derived from petroleum if it looks identical?

Looks of course can be deceiving and here lies a problem.

Many vitamins sold in health shops are synthetic

In fact probably most vitamins are manufactured in factories and usually by the big pharmaceutical companies. This may come as a surprise to many people concerned about their health, but it would be far too expensive to extract all vitamins from natural sources. Most of the companies selling nutritional supplements source the vitamins from pharmaceutical giants and pack and mix them in their individual ways.

Is the mind of man equal to the mind of God/ nature/ millions of years of evolution? Is it possible that the synthetic version has parts missing that cannot be measured and identified by scientists with the tools they have available at present?

Take for example vitamin E. The natural forms are designated d-, as in d-alpha-tocopherol, while the synthetic forms are dl-, as in dl-alpha-tocopherol. The latter is generally used in most research projects because of its cheapness, ready availability and because it is regarded as identical enough. The d-alpha-tocopherol form called 'natural' in the sense that it is bio-identical to the vitamin E found in nature and is derived from various vegetable oils in which high amounts are found. Synthetic vitamin E or dl-alpha-tocopherol is derived from petroleum products and is made up of 8 different fractions of which only one of those fractions is bio-identical to natural vitamin E.

So it is similar but not exact. There is evidence that the body's intelligence does know the difference and will always choose the most natural first as the transport mechanisms are ideally suited to the most natural form of vitamin E. The slight difference in nomenclature points to a difference that should not be disregarded. This can be noticed also in the way polarised light turns when passed through these slightly different molecular structures. The light turns right in the natural from of vitamin E and left in the synthetic.

These small differences may be dismissed by most experts but I regard them as essential details in deciding what supplements to take.

Vitamins are not found in isolation within the food structure. If you could see these vitamins in the food then you would probably notice that they blend in perfectly and are enfolded in a unique way within the plant or food. That particular food in addition would have a range of other nutrients that would complement the action of the vitamin. These 'other' nutrients are called co-factors and enzymes which would allow better absorption and use of the vitamins by the body.

For this reason some companies try to mimic nature and place their synthetic vitamins in a food base to improve absorption and use within the body but in the same way that many of us are suspicious of GMO products which tweak natural products and changes them in subtle ways, we should also be alert to the possible problems that could arise with synthetic vitamins.

Vitamin C is another example of this kind of confusion.

Most containers labelled as Vitamin C contain Ascorbic acid only. Ascorbic acid is only part of the whole Vitamin C complex and while it does seem to be highly active and beneficial in the body and can be used to treat scurvy there may still be subtle and important differences to the whole vitamin C structure as found in the body.

Let your mind imagine the vitamin within the complexity of an orange for example and where the boundary would be between the vitamin C and the rest of the chemical structure. In fact there would be no clear boundaries. The tools and processes we use to separate out chemical structures make it seem as if these chemical structures actually exist in isolation within the body or in food.

What we have identified here is three different modes of vitamin preparations. Firstly there is the vitamin within its food structure that may have been concentrated to increase the quantity of that vitamin or the use of a food item with high quantities of that vitamin. Secondly there is the vitamin synthesised in a laboratory but using natural starting material such as yeast and thirdly a vitamin synthes in the laboratory from a petroleum base material. I don't think anyone would have any trouble deciding which was most natural and which was least natural.

What is natural?

With all these controversies in mind, how is one then to assess what is natural and what is effective? Obviously there are different shades of natural. The most natural are substances, which are grown in their natural environment without fertilisers and are not processed in any way. This would probably tend to exclude many of the substances we regard even as foods and certainly most natural products, which are used to prevent ill health or treat disease.

It is an astonishing fact that in this 'modern' age it is increasingly difficult to buy fruit and vegetables, meat and even fish, which has not been tampered with by modern methods of farming or have not been polluted by the products of industry. Organic farming is about the best we can do to produce wholesome and most natural food products.

It seems that for most of us some kind of compromise is necessary. It is important however that this compromise is a good one, because we are seeing an increase of chronic disease that can no longer be ignored. Foods are not merely nutritional supplements consisting of fats, proteins, carbohydrates, minerals and vitamins, etc.

What is more important is what happens to them within the body. The body in a most miraculous and wonderful way breaks the food substances into its smallest constituent parts so that fats become fatty acids, protein amino acids and carbohydrates are broken down into monosaccharides or simple sugars. These are then absorbed through the intestinal wall and once within the body are converted into hormones, neurotransmitters, enzymes, and all the other chemicals required for the natural function of the body and the replacing of dying cells.

It is important to see this clearly. The foods one eats are the building blocks for every single function, process and substance within the body. Food is hormones. Food is enzymes. Food is immune system. Food is anti-cancer substances. Food is the chemical responses of your emotions. Food moves through your brain in all the myriad processes taking place there. Food is cell, food is liver and heart.

To say that one is one's food is therefore correct. In emphasising the chemical constituents of food one forgets that it is these chemical constituents that eventually become the body. There is a constant flow between the food that one eats and the cells that are being replaced in the body. It is for the above reasons that diet management is of special interest to any practitioner interested in natural health.

- Eating junk food creates a junk body

- Eating processed foods creates a body that is no longer simply natural

- Eating contaminated food contaminates and interferes with normal function within the body.

- Eating food deficient in nutrients means that metabolic processes cannot function normally.

What complicates the discussion of 'natural' is the revolution in processing and packaging and the demand of government, professionals and the public for quality control. None of this was necessary or possible in earlier times. People used what they could get and what was in season and applied their knowledge and experience to the maintenance of health and the treatment of disease. Any discussion about 'what is natural' would make no sense to them.

All this has now changed and the discussion of what is natural takes on a meaningful and even urgent debate. One could become deficient in vitamins and minerals and even ill eating only foods labelled in supermarkets as natural. In general this would not apply to eating fresh fruit, vegetables, meat and fish. Although with the amount of pollution present today and particularly in some countries, even these natural foods are so contaminated with poisons from polluted water, feeds, fertilisers and chemical poisons that the word 'natural' may not exactly apply to these foods.

These factors become urgent and even serious when one considers that the majority of human beings today are no longer receiving sufficient fresh products and are replacing fresh foods with processed foods, which are deficient in vital health promoting substances and even poisoned with colouring matter, preservatives, rancid oils and other by-products such as drug traces, poisonous metal ions, chlorine and fluoride, etc.

It is under these circumstances that the principles of natural medicine become of such importance to everyone concerned with good health and the promotion of good health. One can no longer take for granted that a relatively good diet is sufficient to maintain health. We discuss all this in later chapters and indicate the issues involved and empower everyone to take responsibility for their own health and to take this understanding with them next time they go and see their doctor.

Modern medicine has disempowered the sick individual to such an extent that in general few patients question the fact that doctors are using highly dangerous substances to treat disease, suggest operations which are often unnecessary, are supported by an industry which is enormously biased towards the use of chemicals to treat disease and practitioners who know very little about lifestyle management, diets and natural approaches to health and disease.

What is a 'natural product'?

Natural substances are not merely chemicals strung together into a particular configuration. When oxygen and hydrogen combine to make water something of a miracle takes place. Their individual properties disappear and are replaced not by a combination of their individual properties but something quite unique and different. There is very little in water that would suggest that it is a combination of oxygen and hydrogen and there is also very little in hydrogen and oxygen to suggest that water could arise from their interaction and combination.

When mixtures of elements become a compound something happens to the individual components such that a new level of complexity emerges, new properties develop and the individual goals of the mixture of substances become replaced by a common goal of the new compound.

When a mixture of substances combine to make a compound something is added that is more than the sum of the parts.

One needs in addition to remember that the basic building blocks are particles of energy which also have properties and that all systems are interpenetrated by magnetic fields, electric fields and other energy influences which will influence the system according to the resonance and interaction of forces within the substance.

Matter has physical, electromagnetic and informational components.

The issue here is the complexity of all biological and organic substances. They are not merely mixtures but complex compounds. They are not only chemical but also energetic and carry subtle information. Anything added or subtracted may have subtle or even not so subtle effects on the way the substance interacts within itself and towards the outer environment. If the 'active ingredient' is removed from an herb there should be no surprise if its properties change, in fact one would expect such changes to occur. We could consider for a moment all the changes that may occur:

• The active ingredient may have a much more narrow range of effects.

• The response of the biological system to which it is fed may also vary.

• The so called 'inactives' in the herbal product may be functioning as dampers, controllers, directors, assistants etc. to the active ingredient. Without reins the horse is much more difficult to control. Side effects and other effects may become more obvious and prominent.

• The whole herb is a single intelligence. Something is operating in that herb maintaining its integrity. Molecules communicate via specific electromagnetic waves and chemical signals are present in the herbal structure maintaining a sense of self and function.

For all these reasons removing the active ingredient or changing it in any fundamental way cannot be regarded as perfectly natural and should be handled with great care and respect.The active ingredient is a new product. It may be the loudest and most prominent note within a musical score yet it is not the whole song.

Cutting, removing, splicing, mixing, adjusting, combining, replacing seems to be the way of scientists. It has helped to make the world much more comfortable along the way but when we tamper with living systems great care needs to be taken because of the complexity of the data available and how little we really know about function.

Synthetic vs natural

Science has indeed complicated and even changed the meaning of the word natural. Perhaps the best one can do is try to draw a line somewhere between that which is decidedly synthetic and unnatural and that which is definitely natural. Knowledgeable people will continue to argue where that line should be drawn and it is unlikely that there will ever be a consensus.

What is Natural Medicine?

In the chapters on principles of diet management and supplements for optimum health, I do make an attempt to at least define some principles, which the ordinary person in the street can use to choose a diet which is healthy and nourishing and supplements which will support a healthy lifestyle. The public does need to choose wisely in a marketplace that is often not health promoting but profit orientated.

It seems that I have avoided, in the end, defining the word natural. This should not surprise anyone. Try defining at what point in the dying process is a person truly dead (when the heart stops, the brain is dead or every cell in the body no longer is functioning) or when is the foetus sufficiently well developed to be a human being. These do not have clear and precise answers until it becomes clear and precise. That is to say when there is general agreement with everyone concerned and even then it may just be a concensus statement rather than an absolute truth.

When there is no general agreement then we are in the grey zone, which will always remain the grey zone until other facts become obvious. This is the nature of observation, experience and science although I doubt that grey zones can ever be removed entirely. The more facts we have do not to our surprise remove the confusion or clear the grey zone, but very often only opens other areas of doubt. In this way the grey zone remains just as large although its shape usually changes.

My own personal view is that each company producing a product, which is subject to any process outside its commonly recognised natural state, should justify its claim that the product is natural. The public must then make their own decision whether they wish to buy into that company's products or not.

This book does provide guidelines for making decisions, but in reading the chapter on scientific medicine one begins to recognise the limitations of science in its investigation of biological systems. Modern society has invested science with the intelligence to know eventually everything. Even many scientists believe this to be true and refer to a 'universal field theory', which will allow them to predict and to know everything there is to know about this reality. Quantum Physics has however shown us clearly that it is impossible to know everything .The world is too complex and chaotic. The mystery remains and will keep us busy to the end of time.

Some guidelines to follow in trying to make nutrient choices that are most natural:

• Organic fresh food is generally the best. The emphasis is on 'fresh'. This would include free range chicken and eggs, meat from animals that are also free ranging and not injected with drugs and other chemicals such as growth hormones.

• Cold pressed oils rather than processed oils.

• Rather than using single or combinations of vitamins and minerals choose Superfoods, naturally occurring full-spectrum food extracts containing the complex vitamins and minerals required. These food extracts and concentrates will also have the essential trace minerals, enzymes and co-factors required for good absorption of the vitamins. The quantity of the vitamins may be much less than in the single nutrient but the quality and combination makes up more than adequately for the lower potency.

• There are a few isolated vitamins that I will prescribe or take for myself and sometimes even in high to very high doses. This is based on research and the experience of other Integrative doctors.

• Cheap synthetic vitamin / mineral combinations should not be taken for prolonged periods. Some companies add a concentrated food base to these vitamin/mineral combinations. This is a good idea as it adds other essential nutrients.

• Herbal powders and tinctures should be from organic stock and within the expiry date.

• Any extractions of active ingredients and other manipulation require evidence based research to support their use.

Chapter 2

There is a massive pine tree outside my window perhaps 100 years old. It stands on the side of a farm road that winds its way towards the main road. Wagons pulled by horses must have once upon a time moved past the tree. Men, women, children, cows and goats and perhaps even some wild animals may have passed by the tree and even sat under its shade.

Some days I think about the little seed that germinated, stretched its roots downwards seeking water and nourishment and extended itself upwards to the light and warmth of the sun. I wonder about the stories it could tell and I sometimes listen to its song as the wind and its branches play together.

History of Natural Medicine

History, to a large extent, does depend on the historian. One has only to consider the circumstances of Princess Diana's death to recognise the truth of this. Despite the fact that every effort was made to find the 'truth' of what happened there are still today a number of different versions of that motor car accident that killed the wife of Prince Charles.

My approach to the history of natural medicine must be seen in the same light. It is not the authoritative text on the history of natural medicine, nor is it the only version. It is merely my version to try and clarify some points, which I wish to make so that we can understand together the confusion and conflict that exists in the healing profession today.

Was the Ancient World Primitive and Unsophisticated?

There is a tendency by the average person in most contemporary societies to believe that the modern world is a very far cry from the way the world was thousands of years ago and even perhaps only a century ago. We tend to consider ourselves as very advanced, superior in intellect and sophisticated in our approach to life in general. Thousands of years ago people were primitive, unsophisticated, barbaric and uncivilised.

This is not my viewpoint. The more I study and investigate traditional Chinese medicine and acupuncture, the more respectful I become of this very ancient art and science of medicine. My reading of Traditional Indian medicine and also Tibetan medicine only confirms that we are dealing with a most profound and sophisticated philosophy and a practical approach, which supports this philosophy.

Some textbooks on acupuncture claim that acupuncture points were an accidental and fortuitous discovery. While shooting arrows at each other primitive man discovered that arrows penetrating the body would occasionally relieve painful conditions. It is highly unlikely that this explanation is true. One has only to consider the sophistication of the philosophy that came with acupuncture and the detail and proliferation of supporting facts that accumulated over time.

Let us consider the following observations, which I believe, would dispute any idea that the history of acupuncture was an accidental and haphazard affair. Firstly the points were described in considerable detail as to their location. Not an area but an exact anatomical description, which can often be palpated. Secondly and perhaps even of more importance, each point was described in great detail as to its properties and function. Some points were regarded as minor points with only local effects while other points had major effects far removed from its position.

Stomach 44 for example is a point on the foot, which is often used to treat painful conditions of the head. Many of the observed responses cannot be explained by any present known anatomical or physiological effects. There is a point on the middle of the leg, which will often release a frozen shoulder. A point on the lower arm will treat nausea and another point on the end of the small toe can be used to turn the foetus when presenting as a breech presentation.

Major points have considerable and detailed information as to their anatomical site, ways to stimulate or sedate, how to combine with other points, their influence around the body and their special qualitative effects and difference from other points. All this information was collected and recorded without any scientific tools to measure energy or chemistry.

Similarly in Chinese Herbal Medicine there is a vast library of information on hundreds of herbs. Without knowing any of the chemical ingredients of the herbal substances the ancient herbalists were nevertheless able to record in great detail the properties and effects of the various herbs.

Interestingly also the herbs are categorised in a most unusual way. The herbalists classified the herbs according to the manner in which they were able to move energy in the body/mind system. This information was not based on chemical properties of the plants but rather on the way the plants could promote and harmonise normal function in the body by their 'energetic' influence.

These early investigators had no machines to measure energy and yet seemed familiar with the concept of energy. They were obviously using the word 'energy' to mean something different to that intended by modern scientists. 'Energy' is the usual translation of the Chinese symbol and written in English as 'Qi'.

Qi is more than the energy measured by scientists and incorporates the idea of movement or "that which moves things". It is both the principle of movement and includes also the energy that scientists can measure. Through observation and experience sensitives were able to recognise 'that which can move things', the power within, the dynamics of an inner force of activity.

Most of us have this ability, we talk of good 'vibes' and bad 'vibes', we 'feel' and 'move' according to some inner pressure, we know of 'gut' feeling, we are comfortable or uncomfortable in certain spots, spaces, situations, with certain people, plants, animals etc. Energy is all around us and we are picking up signals and giving off signals.

The same seems to apply to both animate and inanimate things. Even crystals and metals radiate 'energy' and affect us in some way or another. Plants and animals have their own signature tune. It was to this process and 'energy' that ancient practitioners had special knowledge of and experience in. They could 'feel' the 'vibes' of people, animals, plants, crystals, gems and metals.

This Sensitivity is Within us All.

We are making decisions all day based on Unconscious or Conscious Feelings.

This sensitivity can be enhanced & developed.

Much of this is mechanical, conditional and even instinctive. Nevertheless there is also a deeper 'knowing' and intuitive process at work. Herbs are enormously complex structures with a multiplicity of chemical ingredients. From our present knowledge of chemistry one could suggest certain possible actions of these herbs, yet these are only suggestions and may not accord with the herbs' clinical effects when used by practitioners.

Despite very little understanding of chemistry the herbalists of old were able to compile volumes of texts based on experience and that subtle sensitive inner knowing mentioned above. What applies to Chinese traditional medicine is also applicable to all ancient and traditional systems of medicine. All these systems contain vast libraries of information that seemed to have been acquired in this way.

Experience, Intuition and Common Sense

It would be unfair to say that these early practitioners and herbalists did not apply their minds to what they were doing, experience, intuition and common sense was certainly co-ordinated by a good dose of logic and possibly even careful experiment. In this way the writings and texts were generally a careful compilation of human being using all the faculties available to them.

The Tracking Skills of the Bushmen,

Walk About Skills of the Australian Aborigines,

Pyramids in Egypt and Temples in South America.

The tracking skills of the South African Bushmen are well known. The ability of the Australian Aborigines to survive in the arid terrain and find water and food is astonishing and there are also the remarkable building structures such as the pyramids in Egypt and the temples in South America. Again we can recognise the same skills indicated above. Nothing special in a way.

It has always been with us and they belong to each and every human being. It has many names – intuition, gut feeling, feeling with the heart, extra-sensory perception, telepathy, insight, sixth sense, hunch, innate knowledge and even instinct. This potential has always been with us and may have even been much more developed in earlier times. It is a natural, important and even essential inherent capacity of not only the human being, but also all that which lives.

What does seem to be true is that modern man has emphasised the logical and thinking potential of the human brain, while in earlier times when less information was available people had to rely on this sixth sense. If one examines this process carefully then one may become aware that intuitive information has a different character to information derived from thought only. It appears to rise up and become conscious. There is a knowing without thought.

Life is so Complex that Logic Alone would not be Enough to Help us Survive

Logic is slow and cumbersome compared to this other way of knowing, which is generally instantaneous, often surprising and draws in information that has often a transcendental nature. This ability to gain information and function outside thought is common stuff and we would indeed find it very difficult to function without these very wonderful skills.

Driving a motorcar using thought only would be tiresome, slow and even dangerous. This is the way the learner driver begins. In learning to type one goes through the same steps. I have learnt to type with all 10 fingers, but would have difficulty in telling anyone where the letter keys are situated. My fingers seem to know, but please don't bring logic or thought into the process.

This quality is not easy to identify, but certainly the moment thought appears, spontaneity and magic disappears, the system slows down, creativity and insight becomes much less obvious. The moment I think about my typing, I become confused and my creative writing abilities are affected.

What characterised ancient civilizations and men and women of those times is that they had a highly developed 6th sense, an absolute necessity in order to survive the rigours of a society without running water. They had a capacity to know much more than they could possible know using logical thinking only.

As one would expect in any society, there were some men and women with special skills, a greater sensitivity than others. These were the mystics, the saints, the healers, the shamans and sangomas, the medicine men and women. Many of these specially gifted ones were able to investigate these attributes, recognising them as a bridge to a higher source of information. Some used this gift wisely and for the benefit of others while others chose to use these gifts in a selfish, arrogant and greedy way. These latter people were called black magicians.

When I visited China, I met one of the old masters of acupuncture who was regarded as the greatest expert in needle technique. He has written 4 or 5 small textbooks on the art of needle technique only i.e. the way to insert needles into the body in order to produce certain effects. His own teacher was his father.

I was told that for the first few years of his training he followed his father around holding the tray containing the needles. His father hardly spoke to him. This was the traditional way. All teaching was through watching and absorbing as it were the knowledge that was being offered.

This process of learning should not surprise us. Remember that humans needed to communicate with each other, even before language was developed. In her walkabout with the Australian aborigines the author Marlo Morgan (Mutant Message Down Under) describes how they seem to communicate without many words and even without words. There was a 'knowing' what was required and when to prepare for moving or finding food and water.

In the case of the Chinese herbalists this intuitive process was in fact coupled with organised thinking and slowly a body of information accumulated and was written down for students and a future generation of herbalists. In the African tradition there are to my knowledge no written records. African herbalists have teachers who pass on the herbal tradition to them, but in addition use the gift of intuition and sometimes consult with their ancestors through trance states or throwing of the bones. All these techniques are just different ways to facilitate contact with another source of 'knowing'.

So much communication amongst animals is wordless (birds flying in formation) and even with human beings much communication is without words.

It seems that this ability is not much respected today. The person with green fingers, who seems to have a special knowledge of plants, is often less appreciated than the person who has gone through university and obtained honours in Botany. The individual who can 'speak' to animals or dolphins, for example, is much less honoured and respected than the Professor of zoology who may have a great deal of information on those animals, but can't look after a pet.

It is a strange paradox that in ancient times and even today amongst simple people living close to nature, intuition was an essential and respected skill, while in modern societies the intellect, logic, IQ and having a university degree seems more important and serious and considered essential criteria for obtaining jobs and moving up the ladder of success.

Intellect vs Intuition

As we have discussed above, the history of natural medicine is in the end the way human beings have applied their mind to the matter. Before man could even speak, communication was still possible. Animals communicate. Watch the way birds fly in formation or fish swim together. Using a range of sounds animals are able to communicate in quite surprisingly complicated ways. This skill without thought must have been the earliest development of intuition.

Intuition was a survival kit because it gave early human beings information about plants, animals, the earth and the planets and about the nature of life sufficient to allow them to survive and later create the wonders of the world that still holds us in some awe today.

Logic and thinking must have been a later development. Some biologists tend to dismiss these processes as being merely instinctive and therefore mechanical and without any special features. This however denies the incredible dynamism, creativity, purposiveness and even intelligence that seem to be common even in the very lowly life systems.

The history of natural medicine and the development into the modern medicine we have today is therefore a history of the development of man's mind from instinctive and intuitive processes, which emphasised a more natural approach to health and disease to logic and thought and the development of science.

The latter approaches would lead in time to the development of a mechanistic and scientific medicine far removed from the natural medicine of previous centuries. It is not surprising that early humans should have developed intuition to such a remarkable degree. They had no guns to defend themselves, no supermarkets to buy food, no taps with a ready supply of water and no radio or TV to inform them of weather conditions or what the time was. Instead they had to rely on their 6th sense. It was in fact essential for survival.

It is not that today we have lost the skill of intuition, of knowing, of inspiration, that gut feeling that arises and gives warning or direction, it is that another faculty of thought, logic and modern science has come forward to dominate the way we function.

So we leave the history of Natural Medicine recognising that it was the history of man's development of his inner skills that would lead later to the further development of ways of using the brain and especially the left side logical thinking brain, leading in time to scientific progress and the modern world we have today.

Chapter 3

For a moment in time the intensive care room was empty apart from the person I had come to visit. Her face was pale but strong and the breathing slightly laboured. Only yesterday she had been involved in a serious motor car accident and while there were no internal injuries many bones were fractured.

At least three intravenous tubes were attached to her arm and neck and the ticking and clicking of the various machines were the only sounds in the room.

I stood quietly taking in the scene and slowly became aware of another sound. It was the silence itself enveloping and wrapping itself around the contents of the room. My body sighed and a tingling sensation crept up the back of my neck. It seemed that for a moment I heard the sound of angels singing and I knew for the first time that those lying in the intensive care were well protected and cared for.

A History of Modern Medicine

As indicated in the previous chapter on a history of natural medicine, this chapter is only 'a' history of conventional medicine and not 'the' history of conventional medicine. My purpose in this chapter is to indicate the change in thinking which has created the basis upon which the history of modern medicine can be seen in its proper perspective.

The history of modern science perhaps started the moment that Galileo put the first telescope invented to his eye and looked up into the sky at the moon. If we try and imagine that moment in history the poignancy of it is quite remarkable. Keep in mind that up to that moment in time for men and women, heaven was the place of the Gods. Mother Moon, Father Sun, Mars the warring planet, Venus goddess of love, Mercury the messenger of heaven and many others and all the stars had there own mystery and power. In the formation of the clouds one could almost see the gods battling each other or sailing past in pursuit of new goals and tasks.

Suddenly a mere mortal, with the aid of a tool that he had constructed with his own hands, looked up into the sky and announced to the world that the moon was not a god, but only a barren piece of rock full of craters and it was possible therefore that all the other shiny objects in the sky were also physical objects without any spiritual content.

No Gods in Heaven, Only Physical Objects Flying Around

What a let down! What a calamity! In one stroke he had disempowered and emasculated the Church, the priests, the rulers, kings and queens of the time. The mystery of the heavens disappeared. There was only air, rocks and fire. As if that was not enough, Galileo was soon looking down the newly developed microscope and announced that, like the moon, there was no spirit inside the body, but only matter; physical substance in the body and physical matter in the heavens. Bits and pieces of things just like on earth, nothing special. Of course this was exciting news at the time to men and women with an investigative mind, who were fascinated by these discoveries.

The Church however was aghast and dealt with the problem by back peddling as fast as they could go to a new goalpost and came to an agreement with these new masters of the universe. They would keep to spiritual matters and no longer deal with matter. The new scientists could take charge of the material world. This seemed a good compromise. The church would keep out of politics, medicine and any pre-occupation with matter while the scientists could concentrate all their energies on investigating the material world and not bring spirit into the laboratory of science. Everyone was happy.

Separation of Church and State

Attempts were made over the centuries to bring spirit back into matter. The conflict between the vitalists and the materialists is a typical example. The vitalists insisted that there must be some vital substance in matter and especially within living systems. It was this vital substance that was responsible for animation, vitality and vigour within all of life. The materialist poured scorn on this theory.

Vitalists vs Mechanists

- Of what nature was this vital substance?
- Where was it to be found?
- How could it be measured?

The Vitalists could find no answer except to say that it was of such a subtle nature that it could not be measured. Then one day, magnetism was discovered. Suddenly the Vitalists had an answer. Of course the vital substance was magnetic energy. Something that could not be seen yet penetrated through physical matter and could have a controlling influence. Iron filings placed on a flat surface above a magnet would take the shape of the magnetic field.

In a similar manner the cells of the body were held together and controlled by a magnetic field within the body. Magnetism, however, was not to be the holy grail of the Vitalists. Once it could be measured it was no longer outside the ring of science and beyond the reach of the materialist. It now became merely one of the objective features of reality within the ring and an object for investigation by the materialists. The Vitalists were defeated and disappeared as a force.

Another battle was being fought in a stranger setting, which may not seem to have any relationship to that between the Vitalists and the materialists. It was nonetheless as important. The Reformation during the 16th and 17th century was in its own way a battle between two points of view. Christopher Columbus discovered America in 1492 and the world suddenly seemed so much larger. Trade was expanding rapidly and there was a general sense of change and new ideas. The reformation was a religious movement in the Christian Church in Europe, which reflected this new sense of enquiry.

Enter into a Roman Catholic Church and one enters into a museum of art, of light and dark, of stained glass windows, of Saints in every corner and angels flying overhead. Drink of the blood of Christ and rejoice in the singing and communion of spirits shared by all. The Reformation was an attempt to change all this. The leaders of the Reformation regarded the Roman Catholic Church as a remnant of paganism and worship of idols. They wanted to go beyond the form and deal directly with God. The statues were smashed and stain glass windows broken, the incense removed and all vestiges of ceremony banished. The church became bare and austere in keeping with the purity of thought and direct communion required for spiritual contact.

Roman Catholicism vs Protestantism

We will come back to the Roman Catholic Church and the Vitalists, who did have some things in common, but let us for the moment move on in our history of conventional medicine. After Galileo, Descartes represents for me the next milestone in our historic survey of the development of modern science. Descartes is usually regarded as the founder of modern philosophy. He was a brilliant mathematician who was to have a profound effect on the new physics.

He was determined to discover truth and a new way of thinking. To this end he moved into the country in order to be away from all distractions and to apply his mind to these problems. He felt that the human mind alone by the power of its logic and critical application to matters of life and the problems posed by life should be able to resolve these issues. His four postulates, which are discussed in more detail in the next chapter, became the very foundation of the science that was to blossom during the next decades.

Then there was Sir Isaac Newton (1642-1727) regarded as one of the greatest scientists of all time. He is best known for his discovery of the law of universal gravitation and laws of motion. Much of modern science is based on the understanding and use of his laws. As science moved along now very rapidly it seemed that every thing was measurable, that the universe was not haphazard or subject to the whims of the gods. Suddenly the mystery was disappearing and power seem to be flowing in man's direction. With each new discovery light was shining on that, which had been dark for so long. Something most profound was occurring.

The Emergence of Scientific Thinking

The difference between primitive man and modern man, between the vitalists and the materialists, between the Roman Catholic Church and the Protestant Church and between Natural Medicine and Modern Medicine has a commonality, which has within it an important principle which can help us understand what is happening today not only in medicine but also in all human endeavour. Ultimately it is a battle of ideas; ideas that have at their source two modes of functioning. The one mode of function has to do with thought and logic. The other mode of function has to do with intuition and feeling.

Logic and Thought vs Intuition and Feeling

It is of some interest to create a table describing the different manifestations of these two modes of using the mind.

LOGIC	INTUITION
Modern Science	Ancient Science
Uses machines to measure	Uses human sensitivity
Statistics important	Individual important
Cleverness honoured	Wisdom honoured

37

LOGIC	INTUITION
Materialists	Vitalists
Protestant	Roman Catholicism
Science	Art
Left brain	Right brain
Matter	Spirit
Masculine	Feminine
Sun	Moon
Reductionism	Holism
Thought	Feeling

Thought and feeling, logic and intuition are both natural and absolutely normal and useful faculties of all men and women and yet poles apart. There can be no possible way of judging one as being more useful than the other; for when used appropriately both these faculties not only enrich us, but may be critical to life.

When the left-brain denies the existence of the right-brain, when logic insists that feeling is outside reality, then we have a problem. Try driving a motor car using logic/thought only and realise that only beginners drive in this way. Any good driver allows right brain/intuition to operate while keeping the logical mind at attention. If the right brain comes too far forward as it were or wanders off, thinking about yesterday or what needs to be done tomorrow, then attention is lost and poor driving results.

Right Brain vs Left Brain

Modern Medicine has accepted the criteria of Descartes as the basis for its investigation of man. Thus we have a Medicine, which is defined by Science, by logic and statistics, by measurement and by a specialisation in the small and narrow. The whole had to be broken into parts and the power of the human mind as it applies to logic and thought was enough to resolve all problems that would arise.

Modern Medicine Accepts the Scientific Approach to Investigate Human Beings

In the next chapter we will discuss the nature of this science as it developed into the kind of medicine we have today. As its ultimate development scientists postulated a Universal Field Theory that would incorporate all the known laws in the universe. Possessing this mathematical equation would be the Holy Grail of science and would allow man to theoretically have control of the universe. There would be nothing left to discover.

What scientists constantly lose sight of is that what can be measured is only one side of the coin; the left-brain without the right, thought without intuition; human beings with a body, but no spirit and logic without the mystery to sustain and nourish it. The whole is much bigger than what we can possibly comprehend. It is true as Carl Sagan, the passionate advocate of modern science never tires of pointing out, there is a great deal of hocus pocus outside of science.

Certainly this is true and not surprisingly so when one is dealing with mystery, intuition and all those areas in which science has been unable to penetrate. There may be very simple explanations for a host of other 'strange' phenomena. I, however, wish only to point out the remarkable, astonishing and miraculous nature of each of my daily experiences. Anatomy, biochemistry and any other measurement that science comes up with, any formula that science may put together does not in any way come close to explaining or capturing that experience.

Science can only Measure One Side of the Coin of Reality

Carl Sagan has pointed out that science has enlarged man's view and showed us some remarkable and exciting insights into the nature of reality. Certainly he has a point and no one can deny the positive and creative features of science. At the same time, however, science has also debunked a great deal of what I regard as important and sacred and I would like to set the record straight. I do not believe that reality is an open book to science.

There will always be the mystery, immeasurable, enticing and beyond the reach of the tools of science. There are other ways to reach into and measure the mystery however, but to do that does mean leaving the tools of science behind and using and trusting those innate and special abilities that belong to human beings alone; intuition combined with the five senses and an open mind, and so we have made a full circle again.

Would it not be most appropriate and of inestimable benefit to patients if both the intuitive and logic, the traditional way and the way of science were used together to discover the best way to treat health and disease? In the following chapters we will see how in fact this can be done and is being done today.

Chapter 4

When I was 14 years old my mother bought me a microscope and I would spend hours examining the head of a fly, an ant, a grasshopper's leg and other interesting living insects that I could find in the garden. There is such a fascination in breaking things up and looking inside as if this takes one deeper and deeper into the way everything works. Almost 60 years later I realise that I am more interested in what holds it all together and why despite the fact that all matter is made up of a few basic building blocks there is such an enormous variety of expressions.

What is Scientific Medicine?

Evidence tends to be equated with the philosophy of reductionism. Reductionism is a belief that complex data can be reduced to seemingly equivalent simple ones. Its polar opposite is Holism.

Holism is a theory that the universe and especially living nature is correctly seen in terms of interacting wholes (as of living organisms) that are more than the mere sum of their parts. There is a very important difference here, which dictates the way practitioners of these two different philosophies (Holism and medical reductionism) approach the problem of health and disease. Modern medicine has certainly chosen the way of science(breaking things into parts) in its more narrow sense to reflect its approach to health and disease whereas Natural Medicine has always tended to be Holistic in its approach.

Definitions

Holism:

'A theory that the universe and especially living nature is correctly seen in terms of interacting wholes (as of living organisms) that are more than the mere sum of elementary particles.'

Reductionism:

'A belief that complex data etc. can be reduced to seemingly equivalent simple ones.' Collins dictionary

As indicated in the history of modern medicine a process was started by Descartes to break things into smaller and smaller parts in order to understand how these parts worked in the context of the whole. Natural Medicine on the other hand maintained a perspective of wholeness, of relationship, of the interaction between wholes and of an understanding that breaking the whole would change the way it functioned.

The whole was more important than the sum of the parts and a different approach to investigation was required in which the whole was 'teased open' rather than broken apart in order to gain information . The process of opening is somewhat akin to teasing open the weave of a piece of material so that its pattern is not lost, rather than examining a strand which has been removed.

Teasing Open Rather than Cutting up into Pieces

Modern Medicine has often been referred to as scientific medicine while Natural Medicine and its modern equivalent is often referred to as Holistic Medicine or Integrative Medicine. The spelling of holistic without the "w" is in deference to General Smuts one of the great South African political leaders, great philosopher and one of the founders of the World Health Organization (WHO) who in 1926 first published his book *Holism and Evolution*.

One of my favourite quotes taken from his book is the following:

'In its analytic pursuit of parts, science has missed the whole, and thus tended to reduce the world to dead aggregations rather than to the real living wholes which make up nature.' J.C. Smuts.

In this chapter we will consider the mechanism and philosophy of science and compare it to the philosophy of Holism. It is important to keep in mind that like most things, it is the interpretation that makes the difference. It is the interpretation of the Bible in so many different ways that has been responsible for the many different Christian sects. It is the interpretation of 'the law' that can either create a destructive narrow-minded approach to governing with restrictions on individual rights or a creative liberal approach with freedom of creative expression for the individual.

Similarly scientific thinking may be very narrow minded or creative.

Science becomes narrow minded when those members within its community who regard themselves as its protectors insist on defining science in a most limiting way often referred to as 'scientism' rather than good science. In this narrow minded scientific approach, medical journals will only publish articles which agree with their particular paradigm and point of view. Money for research which is supported mainly by pharmaceutical companies will only be directed towards research which supports the present biochemical drug based viewpoint of treating disease which is good for pharmaceutical business and medical education follows the same limited and narrow minded approach. If education follows that bias and does not allow for other viewpoints, it does not further the progress of medicine and is not good science.

Doctors who try to be innovative and use non-pharmacological medicines such as herbs and techniques such as acupuncture, which fall outside the acceptable scientific medical boundaries, are harassed, hounded and their right to practice limited or even stopped.

Only conventional medical oncologists for example are permitted to claim that they treat cancer. Anyone else claiming to treat cancer in other than conventional ways may be subject to the most intimidating methods of harassment. In America for example many of these innovative doctors have been raided by the FDA, taken to court for lengthy and expensive legal battles and had equipment and important papers confiscated.

This has been happening despite the fact that cancer therapy in the majority of cancers is still experimental, new therapies and new combinations of therapies of highly poisonous substances are being used on human beings without knowledge of the long term effects and despite the fact that the real cure rate of cancers has not risen dramatically. Most of these chemical treatments are themselves carcinogenic.

While conventional doctors are able to carry on research with these poisonous substances, other doctors attempting to treat cancer in non-toxic creative ways are invariably intimidated and harassed. This I believe is an abuse of the scientific spirit. Even bills to try to introduce innovative natural cancer treatments to terminal cancer patients with their permission have run into serious objections.

Narrow Minded Science vs A Rich Enquiring Innovative Science

The problem is that the concept of "reductionism" has come to epitomise science and the scientific method while 'Holism' is often regarded as anti-science because of its emphasis on many aspects of life which are mystical and non measurable. What perhaps is forgotten is that the process involved in reductionism is only one of the ways that human beings have investigated the world around them.

Breaking things apart and putting them back together again are all the ways men, women and even children have used to investigate the world, but perhaps the most common way has been observation and experience. Observation of nature in its natural setting and through this contact coupled with a heightened sensitivity and clear thinking is how early human beings learnt how to find water and food, hunt, relate to each other, build shelters and all those myriad things necessary to live and survive.

It was however the development of the scientific method as suggested by Descartes in 1637, which initiated the more limited view of investigation. This approach has become so powerful that it has dominated the history of man in recent times. Science has been used to create machines of destruction to defend and dominate, it has changed the way agriculture is practised, it has brought pollution and modern medicines, electricity and motor cars, high rise buildings and microwaves, but more particularly it has changed the way people think about themselves and the way they deal with life in general.

Not all this is bad of course, and few want to return to the pre-scientific age, but there is perhaps a sense that science or the way we think about science requires a review before it destroys all that we regard as precious and beautiful.

The March of Science

René Descartes, born in France in March 1596, is often regarded as the father of modern philosophy. He studied law and mathematics and this strengthened his own innate tendency towards a respect for logic and rational thinking.

He fled to the country where in the silence of nature he could contemplate the workings of the universe and where he believed he could through the power of logic and reason discover the mechanical principles governing all natural phenomena in one single system.

During the years he spent in the country he developed the following four essentials of the scientific method:

- Accepting only what is clear in the mind.

- Breaking down large problems into smaller ones.

- Arguing from the simple to the complex.

- Checking.

These essentials of Descartes were the early stirring of the scientific method, which led to the following approaches over the subsequent centuries:

- Accepting only what is clear in the mind refers to *Reason* and *Logic*.

- Reason and logic was the background mind set for the development of Mathematics and Statistics.

- Breaking down large problems into smaller ones is the process of Reductionism referred to earlier.

- Arguing from the simple to the complex is the process in which one tries to understand complex systems from a study of their more simple parts.

- Checking suggests the idea that systems are stable and if investigated in the same way under similar conditions in different parts of the world will produce the same results i.e. the scientific method is *Reproducible* anywhere in the world and provided that all the standards are maintained the end result should be the same.

The four Essentials of Descartes have come a long way and have been the powerhouse driving the scientific method today.

Modern science now stands on the following pillars:

- Reductionism.

- Simplicity.

- Reproducibility.

- Logic.

- Prediction.

I would like to use the method of Descartes i.e. logic and reason to consider whether the above approaches are sufficient to examine complex biological systems such as human beings. It must be obvious to anyone who considers the enormous benefits of modern medicine that the scientific method as used today is relevant and is valuable. What we need to consider is whether it is enough and what are its limits when applied to living systems rather than machines.

Reductionism and Simplicity

"A belief that complex data etc. can be reduced to seemingly equivalent simple ones."

The question one needs to ask is whether the simple parts are representative of the whole. That great Holist General Smuts as mentioned above, stated clearly that in breaking things apart the whole was reduced to dead aggregations and that this did not represent in any way the whole. It is a nice idea to think that complex biological systems are similar to complex machines, especially today when the complexity of machines is enormous and beyond most people's understanding and comprehension.

These machines are all built up of small parts. Added together they make up a very complex machine, which is able to perform a large variety of tasks. Such a machine can be broken down and built up again. It can be taken apart and shipped anywhere in the world and provided it is assembled correctly will work again in the same way as before.

Is this true of complex living biological systems? Are they made up of simple molecules strung together and can they be broken apart and the parts examined in order to understand how they function as one whole? This is a very important consideration because it is the very foundation of modern medicine and the way human beings are investigated. This problem is also at the heart of the way we as human being think about others and ourselves and the way we deal with life.

Consider the following two statements and decide which one you believe is closest to the truth:

• Human beings are spiritual beings that have crystallised matter around themselves.

• Human beings are made up of simple elements that over time have learnt how to think.

So are we basically spiritual beings who have passed through the veil of forgetfulness into the physical world of matter or are we just a collection of chemicals that through a process of evolution have arrived at the state of development we have today? What is your choice?

Most of us probably feel very paradoxical about this decision and would like to add 'buts' and 'ifs' and it's not so simple. The point I wish to make is that the answer is indeed complex and may not be either but something of both. Many modern scientists would perhaps refer to this problem as 'upward causation' and 'downward causation'. The idea being that there are higher levels or dimensions which can influence lower levels. Examples could be mind affecting body or energy influencing matter.

The Chinese philosophy of the Tao suggests that the Great Mystery took the substances of the earth and made a vessel from these elements into which He poured Spirit. Thus he made the human being. Jesus also referred to man's dual nature 'Flesh can give birth only to flesh; it is spirit that gives birth to spirit.' Science, one must understand however, does have a very clear point of view and it is this clear point of view that dictates the way medical students are taught and the kind of research and treatment carried out by the conventional medical model.

I was standing one day in the airport chatting to a Professor of Pharmacology about the training of medical students today and his immediate answer was that the bottom line is science and more science. When I suggested that science was not enough to understand human beings and that to understand my wife or child I did not need any science he seemed at first perplexed. Science is good and valuable when applied to those things that can be measured. It is of little value when applied to those things that cannot be measured or where measurement is inappropriate.

Reductionism is a point of view. It is one way only of investigating life. I may have another point of view and you may have a third point of view. The more points of view the better the view. That is not however the way most people and even the average scientist thinks. It is a great sadness that we kill each other for having different viewpoints. The More Points of View, the Better the View

Mixtures vs Compounds

There is an interesting difference between a mixture and a compound. In a mixture each constituent part maintains its own integrity and can be separated from the other elements in the mixture.

In a compound something very strange happens. Each individual chemical gives up its own particular identity to create something new and unique. This new substance has properties which are surprisingly different from its constituent parts. Many if not most of these properties could not be predicted from knowledge of the parts only.

Water is a most unique material. Scientists however would be hard pressed to predict from examining hydrogen and oxygen only all the possible properties of water. Something very special and mysterious happens when hydrogen and oxygen combine together to form water.

If one manages to separate the constituent parts of water into hydrogen and oxygen then all the properties of water disappear and one is left only with the separate properties of oxygen and hydrogen. It is not possible to examine water except as water. The moment any attempt is made to separate a compound into its constituent parts then that compound disappears as a whole functioning unit and one is left with a mixture of substances with its own individual properties.

It is essential to understand this. Mixtures are not compound and compounds become mixtures or bits and pieces of the original compound when broken down or cut apart or separated from the whole. If we consider complex biological systems like plants, animals and especially human beings then we need to keep in mind that these systems are not mixtures of individual elements, but rather highly complex molecular/energetic structures that are able to recreate themselves over and over again.

The reductionistic approach has perhaps deceived us into thinking that biological systems are like complex machines and made up of parts, which can be replaced when broken and repaired if damaged. This image is sustained by a system of medicine which tends to honour the specialist above the general practitioner, the surgeon above the physician, with different departments for each organ system and treats the part rather than the whole person and removes organs and which replaces them where possible.

It seems true that on one level the human being can be dealt with as made up of parts. Hip joints can be replaced, plastic heart valves can be inserted, uteruses can be removed and lens implants can help blind people see again. All this is true and much more. There is no denying the power of the reductionistic approach.

I do not wish to refute this but only to point out that this approach is only one side of the coin and for that reason despite the billions of dollars poured into research, real cancer cures are not around the corner, blood pressure may be controlled but not cured, eczema may be suppressed with cortisone but not healed, rheumatoid arthritis may be treated symptomatically but we are not any closer to producing a real cure for these diseases and most other afflictions of modern man.

Symptomatic treatment may relieve symptoms and signs but they often do this at an enormous expense to the patient in terms of side effects and cost. Almost 100,000 people develop bleeding in the intestinal tract from anti-inflammatory drugs in the USA each year and 10,000 - 20,000 of these patients die. It is said that the benefits outweigh the risks. If these large numbers of deaths are true then should we not be looking for more appropriate natural ways to treat disease rather than high-risk drugs?

Human beings and other biological systems are not simple. Reducing them to simple substances removes the magic, often destroys the life. Everything on this planet is composed of the same simple elements.   Gold and coal are even composed of exactly the same element- carbon, yet how different they are. It seems that something is added each time elements are combined together that science cannot yet measure and perhaps never will.

Science and the reductionistic approach can measure parts of the structure, but provides very little information about the uniqueness of biological systems and what exactly happens to mixtures when they become compounds.   The quantity can be measured, but the qualitative differentiation, which characterizes living systems and in fact even non-living systems, remains a mystery. It is that which is added when molecules are combined together and that which disappears when complex living systems are broken down, which is so interesting and seems to 'slip through our fingers' when subject to the scientific method. It is that which slips through our fingers, which makes all the difference.

Human beings are compounds and not merely mixtures of various elements. It is for this reason that the reductionistic approach when applied to humans will always give limited answers and why the methods of investigation of the ancients must be revisited and respected.

Reproducibility, Logic and Prediction

This is another cornerstone of the scientific method. In order to do any research it is necessary to be able to reproduce the results over and over again and in different laboratories. It is this condition of reproducibility that makes statistics and prediction possible. Reproducibility suggests that there is some logic and order not only in the reductionistic research process but in living systems. In other words living systems have an inner stability and follow laws which make their action predictable.

In 1960 Lorenz, a Meteorologist in America was investigating weather prediction tables and came to the conclusion that absolute weather prediction was impossible for the simple reason that so many factors were involved. He also pointed out that weather patterns, but also other living systems are so sensitive that even small and subtle changes could affect these systems.

This sensitivity of complex systems has become known as the butterfly effect; a butterfly flapping its wings in New York can cause a storm in San Francisco; a small effect creating an enormous response.

What has become clear is that even with the most sophisticated equipment weather forecasting could not become much better than it is today and that the further ahead one attempts to predict the weather the less accurate it is likely to be. Why is this so?

The truth is that firstly complex systems are indeed complex and secondly complex systems found in nature are not separate and isolated from the surrounding space but are open systems connected to other systems and responding continuously to the constant flow and ebb of nature. We will be discussing the nature of systems in a later chapter because it is a fundamental difference in the way conventional medicine and holistic medicine and natural medicine views health and disease. There is no doubt some order in the universe, and scientists are dependent on laws to guide their space ships to the moon and other planets but in a sense this is the easy stuff of science.

There are risks of course and the unpredictable is always there but clever scientists can reduce this risk substantially. Biological systems are however much more complex. It is not that they are outside law. Remember Einstein's cry that God does not play dice with the Universe. It is just that they are so complex and linked to other complex systems that the way any biological system will react or respond to any stimulus is generally not predictable.

It is in fact the special nature of biological systems, which are living systems, that makes them different to billiard balls flying around a table or the planets moving around their orbit. Seeds from the same flower planted on different days will not grow in exactly the same way even though planted in the same soil. The seeds are responding to the environment in ways that are unpredictable to science. My old gardener was a great deal wiser and grew better and healthier plants than the average homeowner using books and advice from experts.

One needs to clearly differentiate between non-living systems, which are moved by forces such as gravity and obey the second law of thermodynamics and living systems, which also seem to be affected by some of these laws but have their own unique set of natural laws and have the ability to make choices within the confines of these laws. We will be dealing with this in more detail in other chapters. It is of some importance to understand how living systems respond in principle even if it is not always possible to predict exactly what will happen.

Conventional Medicine has chosen the methods of science to investigate human beings. This approach has made possible a very fundamental and deep understanding of the physical body of human beings. The strength of this approach has tended to blind scientists to the limitation of this method of investigation and they will often exclude new and innovative approaches just because they follow a different mind set or paradigm. Scientific medicine is only one way to investigate human beings. It is a viewpoint but not the only view.

Scientists generally believe that they need to move from the known to the unknown. They believe that the unknown cannot be known except through investigation with the tools of science. This belief is based firstly on the assumption that everything in the universe eventually must be measurable and secondly that what one already knows is good enough as a starting point to investigate the unknown.

Everything in the Universe is Measurable

Is this true?

Measuring Tools already in use are Good Enough to Measure the Unknown

Is this true?

The belief that everything in the universe is measurable may be very wide off the mark. It assumes that in the end God/Consciousness/quantum space is a mathematical formula, that all human experience and consciousness itself will be clearly definable and measurable, that spirit, soul, willpower, love etc. will either become measurable or shown not to be real but just the puff of smoke emitted from the fire of burning wood.

Science assumes that the tools it uses can journey into the unkown and finally discover the nature of the mystery. There is I believe a huge misconception here. The problem with investigating tools is that they do not so much discover new territory but tend to define the new territory according to their own limitation. This may at first glance be difficult to understand. So let's go slowly through this idea.

- Does looking through blue glass create a blue reality or is the reality blue?

- Pushing meat through a sausage machine creates sausages.

- Passing light through a prism creates colour.

- Biochemists discover the world as bio-chemistry

- Bio-engineers discover the world as electromagnetic.

So do the tools used by scientists to investigate the world show us the world as it is or as the tool being used shapes the world. The biochemists using biochemical tools will identify a reality based on biochemistry and the engineer using the tools of his trade will identify a reality based on electromagnetism. They are clearly right and wrong at the same time. Right because that is what they measure and wrong because it is not the whole story. Without knowing the whole story we can never be absolutely right or know the absolute truth if that is at all possible.

What if the 'unknown' is not biochemical and also outside electro-magnetism as we know it, what then?

What if the tools required to investigate the unknown are the human senses, intuition, thoughts and feelings and not more sensitive machines which can only measure their own limitations? Then perhaps the way of the ancients, of experience and the heart are valid expressions and ways to investigate the very heart of life itself.

What science describes is all that it can know using the tools of science. These tools are extremely useful but always limited. The tools that human beings have which include their senses, intuition, feeling and thinking have emerged out of the evolutionary process and therefore have a sympathetic resonance with the past and the present in a way that scientific tools cannot have. It is for this reason that the experience of practitioners and their patients is valid and needs to be listened to carefully.

Each person, each patient has a valid and valuable insight into their own problem and process. Scientific medicine has tended to dismiss the valuable insights of patients and the experience of practitioners outside the conventional model of medicine. It is time for others to capture the high ground as well and show that there are other ways to investigate nature. It has to do with experience, with self discovery, with a sensitivity and listening ear to nature and especially with a deep respect for the spirit within all things.

Chapter 5

I have always been fascinated by names and the words we use to describe things. The names and the words are just that... names and words; nothing more nor less. We give them meaning and decorate them with our colours of life. The trouble is that the same word can mean different things to different people.

Definitions

The public is bombarded with new therapies daily all advertised as being alternative, complementary, energetic, holistic, natural or just new therapy. For the uninitiated it is often difficult to decide where to go, what to expect and whether the new treatment is just duplicating a treatment one has had before.

The problem is compounded by the fact that therapists and doctors themselves are not clear what their colleagues are doing and why the technique in question may work. We are entering an age of enormous creativity. A new box of tricks has been opened and a whole host of new ideas are emerging, which will in time impinge themselves right into the centre of medical therapeutics and certainly change the very philosophy and principles of medicine.

This chapter will be divided into two parts. In the first section we will deal with the broad categories in which the different therapies fall while in the second section I will discuss some of the therapies separately. This book is about philosophy and principles and what is common to all therapies. The therapies I have chosen to discuss are the most popular and help to highlight the different approaches. They are not discussed in detail as there are many books in which more information can be obtained.

Broad Categories of Natural Medicine

Manipulative

This is a hands on approach and usually consists of the therapist massaging, touching, rubbing, shaping or manipulating the soft tissue or adjusting the bones and joints according to very clearly defined techniques. There are now such a multitude of techniques that some observers may be prepared to dismiss all of them as being mumbo jumbo.

This is a hasty and unfair judgement as the variety merely confirms the enormous and creative potential of human beings. Touching the body in a kind and caring way always produces positive results. Even the hand on the shoulder as a person leaves the office can make all the difference to a consultation.

In this group we can include the chiropractor and osteopath, massage therapist, physiotherapists, reflexology, Rolfing, Bowen technique, Cranio-sacral and all the other hands on procedures used by practitioners and therapists. It is important to recognise that each one of these professions generally does not consider its practice as manipulation or massage only.

There is a holistic and even spiritual dimension to many of the techniques. The part of the body that is being touched, massaged or manipulated is connected to the whole person (body/emotions/ mind/spirit) so that any correction in one part of the body will be reflected eventually in the whole body-mind system. In other chapters this will be explored more fully.

The different techniques reflect the multilayered, holographic web, which constitutes the human physical frame and its energetic components. The image of a record player comes to mind. There are many ways to improve the quality of the sound by physically changing some of the component parts or playing around with the numerous knobs on the machine until the sound is perfectly to one's satisfaction.

One can do exactly the same with the human being out of harmony or diseased. One can move the component parts or find ways to change the flow in which the soft tissue and bones move and the energetics of the system is co-ordinated.

What is remarkable is how very often small adjustments can have major effects which seem to penetrate into the heart of the system. The results are often miraculous and long lasting. As one begins to understand the nature of natural healing and the dynamics of what one is working with, these results become under- standable in principle even if the actual mechanism remains mysterious. I don't think that one system is better than another, only that one practitioner may be better suited to your needs.

Naturopathic and nutritional medical approaches

This branch of medicine includes all forms of water therapy, fasting and diets, enemas, compresses, herbs, exercise and in nutritional medicine includes the use of vitamins, minerals and other supplements.

The general aim of this approach is to encourage the body to heal itself by what is referred to as cleansing, detoxification and nutritional supplements.

Energy medicine

This is a diverse group of healing approaches and includes acupuncture, spiritual healing, homoeopathy, flower remedies, colour therapy, light therapy, low energy laser light therapy, Bicom, Vega, Quantum Xeroid, Rife, Radiesthesia and radionics, Sound therapy and many others. The basic tenet of this type of therapy is that behind the biochemical and physiological processes is an energetic template and that by adjusting this energetic template changes will become apparent in the biochemistry and even the anatomy.

The image would be that of a magnet with its magnetic field. If a piece of paper sprinkled with iron filings is placed over the magnet then the iron filings will arrange themselves in a pattern according to the shape of the magnetic field. Moving the iron filings around would be equivalent to trying to adjust the biochemistry with drugs, which work for some hours only. By changing the magnetic field the iron filings will move spontaneously and without effort.

Energy medicine attempts to change the energetics and thus influence the physicality. Does energy exist in the body? Where it is and why doctors do not know more about energy will be discussed in later chapters.

Moving an Ohmeter which measures electrical fields over the body will demonstrate clearly that the body also has electromagnetic fields. The ECG and EEG are electrical recordings of the heart and brain. It is an assumption that these fields have nothing to do with health and disease and that their only interest to doctors is to measure heart and brain activity. So why has there been so little research in this area of medicine? Suffice perhaps to say at this point that pharmaceutical companies with all the money for research are not interested in investigating anything to do with energy.

Like the colours of the spectrum, which have a range of frequencies, so too one finds in energy medicine many contrasting therapies and approaches. The colour red is heating and the colour blue is cooling. Energy medicine by using energetics in different ways has created many different modalities of use from colour to sound to acupuncture and laying on of hands. This is a wide open field of creative research and expect to see many new and useful ideas emerging from this field of interest.

Psycho-spiritual approaches

In this category one can include the following: Hypnosis, NLP (neuro-linguistic processing), PNI (psychoneuro-immunology), rebirthing, regressing, repatterning and many other psychotherapeutic approaches and including many of the techniques used by Sangomas and Shamans.

These approaches have to do with mind over matter , visualisation, positive affirmation, ceremony and even prayer. In the psycho-spiritual approaches the 'mind' is clearly involved and is the focus of attention. In energy medicine, it is the energy that is the focus of the attention. In the psycho-spiritual approach the mind is involved and the intention to make a shift in consciousness. I call this the 'informational' shifting group.

Principle guidelines of classification:

The above groups all use one or a combination of three approaches:

- Physical: body work

- Energetic: electromagnetic

- Informational: mind-consciousness

Very few of the various modalities use only one of the above modalities consciously or unconsciously. The massage therapist may be only concerned about relaxing muscles and getting rid of knots but just being close to someone and having hands on that person will also involve a sharing of electromagnetic energy and information through that contact.

A Guide to Some Therapies

Conventional Medicine (also Orthodox Medicine or Allopathic Medicine):

This is not a 'Natural medicine' approach but needs to be included in order to make some sense of the approaches regarded as natural.

Conventional medicine is the generally accepted approach by the medical establishment to health and disease. This approach has developed out of the Newtonian/Cartesian understanding, which has been the basis of modern science until very recent times. This is the so-called 'scientific approach' which as indicated in chapter 3 and 4 has developed a number of very simple assumptions:

- Firstly, that all complicated structures are derived from very simple underlying building blocks.

- That by dividing these complicated structures again and again, one comes closer and closer to these fundamental building blocks and that studying these fundamental blocks will lead to an understanding of the complex whole.

- That for every effect there is a preceding cause.

- That for every cause there is a predictable effect, which can be calculated.

From this model we have ended up with a view of human beings made up of cells through which biochemistry flows. It is the concentration on biochemistry which has lead to the development of drugs and the growth of pharmaceutical companies.

The view of the human being as a body made up of parts has seen the growth of surgery and surgeons who are the mechanics moving and cutting the parts in order to arrange the parts in different ways or 'fix' the part according to this mechanical understanding of the body parts.

We understand today that these assumptions are an enormous over-simplification when one is dealing with living systems. These approaches were developed by scientists who had physical structures in mind. They understood the way machines were made and assumed that somehow everything in the universe was made in the same way.

This idea was supported by the fact that it seemed that in the beginning of creation very simple elements were present in the form of hydrogen, nitrogen and oxygen. From these very simple beginnings it was assumed all the complex forms of life eventually resulted.

This was a nice idea and its simplicity appealed to everyone and it is in fact still the dominant theory recognised by most scientists.

Living systems however are not machines made up of parts which can be taken apart and put together again much like a child constructs something with building blocks or Lego. Any attempt to do this with living systems will however create enormous problems and possibly even kill that life form.

It seems that life is not just a collection of bits and pieces strung together. Something is added that is much more that the sum of the parts. It is as if in putting the machine together a fundamental change happens so that the machine becomes much more than what would seem possible from the knowledge one has of its constituent parts.

The scientific model of breaking things into parts will always have limited value. Other systems of medicine have recognised the special nature of the whole. One begins to recognise that as these simple elements, which constitute matter, combine together in more and more intricate ways that new emerging properties appear.

Traditional systems of medicine believed that the physical nature of living systems was drawn from the earth while its spiritual nature came from the heavens. In other words that which was added to the physical, which made it much more than the sum of parts, was spirit or some special vital substance. It was this spirit or vital substance which bound the parts together in a unique way and was responsible for these emerging properties, which do not seem to be intrinsic to the simple elements which make up matter. Heaven and earth were thus united in all living substances.

Holistic Medicine:

Within the philosophy of Holistic medicine is the idea that in order to understand the whole one must examine it as a whole and not in little pieces. The whole is a system of interconnected processes. Professor George Jaros, one of our great systems theorists said of systems that examining a system was like examining a tapestry. There was the overall picture but sometimes it was necessary to open up the weave in order to understand its basic structure better. Cutting the tapestry into pieces not only destroyed the picture but also the construction of the tapestry.

The Holistic practitioner always understands that a human being is a body/emotions/mind/spirit entity, that this complex entity functions as one whole and therefore any part of the system is always in contact with the whole. Mind affects body and body affects mind. Emotions affect mind and mind affects emotions. Pain in body affects emotions, affects mind etcetera.

Biological systems are open systems – open outwardly to the environment and inwardly to the world of spirit. It is this openness which more than any other property differentiates biological living systems from relatively closed non-living systems. We breath out carbon dioxide and trees use the carbon dioxide and provide us with oxygen. In a certain sense the trees are part of our lung system.

Holistic practitioners believe that the human system always functions as one piece and therefore understand that all the symptoms and signs are merely expressions of one underlying disharmony within the system and not expressions of different 'diseases'. Hypertension, gout and diabetes within one person are all the result of an underlying disharmony within the body-mind system and this disharmony needs to be treated rather than the end points. Conventional doctors would regard hypertension, gout and diabetes as three separate diseases and the patient may even be treated by three different specialists. Holistic doctors would regard these three conditions as the result of an underlying combination of dysfunctions expressing themselves outwardly in these three ways.

Holistic medicine was the early stirrings which slowly gathered momentum and developed later into what is now called Integrative Medicine. (see below)

Complementary and Alternative Medicine (CAMS):

CAMS Medicine today is generally understood to mean all forms of natural approaches to ill health which are not conventional medicine. The focus tends to be on supporting health and allowing the body's own innate intelligence to do the work of healing. So this approach is an 'alternative' approach and 'complements' the body's healing processes by supporting, activating and nourishing the body.

This is a broad category and includes homeopathy, herbal medicine, aromatherapy, Body Talk, osteopathy, chiropractic and all the other systems of healing with many diverse names using natural approaches to stimulate healing.

Integrated Medicine:

Medical doctors are spreading their wings and learning acupuncture, homeopathy, various forms of manipulation and many other forms of natural healing systems. More and more doctors are integrating various forms of new philosophies and techniques. This however does not only apply to medical doctors but also to most other health professionals.

Chiropractors are mixing their classic manipulation techniques with many other forms of non-manipulative techniques such as body alignment, trigger point and pressure point applications combined often with muscle testing. Physiotherapists are also mixing their classic approaches with acupuncture, dry needling, laser therapy and many other non-classical techniques.

Naturopaths, homeopaths and most other practitioners are all integrating various old and new ideas into their practices. The boundaries between professionals are becoming less clear and professional jealousy and acrimony becomes an increasing problem. Some governments are suggesting that professionals must clearly define their scope of practice in order to prevent this mixing.

Integration is however a reality that must be faced and dealt with in a creative way so that the patients are the winners. I am seeing an enormous amount of creativity emerging out of this mixing process and I believe that it is basically good. While some controls may be necessary to prevent harm to patients from badly trained practitioners this mixing process is part of the natural evolution of what I expect to be a new kind of medicine.

Integration is also happening in the way practitioners are starting to work together. There are today group practices in which a number of practitioners with different expertise come together to share information and give clients better options. Medical doctors, acupuncturists, physiotherapists, aroma- therapists, etc. all working together under one roof and often coming together to discuss common problems. Integrated medicine is here to stay and what is alternative and unusual will become commonplace within the next few years.

Integrative Medicine is an emerging medicine. Its principles and practice are in the process of being defined and structured. It needs to be left to float free still and I believe it will become the conventional medicine of the future.

Of special note is the way medical practitioners are dealing with this integration and pushing the edges of the conventional paradigm or model. These Integrative doctors tend to emphasise lifestyle changes, supporting health and dealing with the disease if appropriate. I cover more details of this approach in the rest of this book.

Orthomolecular Medicine:

This is an approach to the treatment and prevention of disease by adjustment of the chemical constituents of the body primarily by nutritional management. By the use of a chemical free and low sugar diet combined with high doses of vitamins and minerals cures are produced. Doses of nutritional supplements are often much higher than the recommended daily dose and some expertise is therefore required at these high doses.

Professor Pauling, who was a recipient of a Nobel prize for Medicine, was one of the best know Orthomolecular physicians and was responsible for making the use of high doses of Vitamin C popular. Dr Hoffer in Canada has used very high doses of Vitamin B3 to treat Schizophrenia and to lower cholesterol.

Natural medicine cannot however, be patented and this accounts for the fact that its use in treating disease has not been extensively researched or publicised widely. Pharmaceutical companies have the money to finance research and especially to advertise widely. Drugs can be patented. It is not surprising therefore that natural medicines are generally not well known to medical doctors and tend to be regarded as 'soft' without any real therapeutic value in the treatment of disease.

Anthroposophical Medicine:

This is the system of medicine that developed from the research, writings and teachings of Rudolph Steiner. The system of medicine is based on his philosophy and incorporates a view of man as a three fold being with equal status given to body, soul and spirit.

The system is Holistic and incorporates the use of herbal and homeopathic medicines together with sound and music therapy. The medicines are prepared from plants grown according to the suggestions of Rudolph Steiner and processed in a very special way in order to bring out the special potential required from the combination used.

Homeopathic Medicine:

Developed by Heinemann this medicine is of relatively recent origin. Most conventional medical doctors and scientists generally dismiss it as quackery in the extreme despite the fact that it is being used today by thousands of medical and non-medical practitioners throughout the world. The reason for this scepticism has to do with the way these medicines are prepared. It requires a process of diluting and shaking, which is repeated many times.

Homeopaths regard the most dilute remedies as the most powerful and deep acting. This flies in the face of modern science that diluting a substance should give it a broader and deeper action. That it should have any action at all seems indeed remarkable yet that is the experience of all those who use homeopathic remedies. In the higher dilutions all traces of the original substance disappear and one seems to be left only with the diluting substance, which is usually alcohol. Something very strange indeed seems to be going on here. Are the claims of healing nothing more than placebo effects or spontaneous remissions?

As is usual in these circumstances all the criticism and cries of quackery come from those who have never practised this form of healing and think they know better. Certainly this phenomenon appears to be outside the present known laws of science but then science has not yet been able to measure emotions, mind and spirit or understand the energetics (electrical, magnetic, subtle) operating within the body.

This is a most unprofessional, biased and unscientific point of view. Any practitioner using homeopathy on a regular basis very soon becomes convinced of the efficacy of these remedies and is not particularly concerned that its mechanism of action is not known. This is not especially unusual.

Electricity, gravity, the exact action of aspirin, the movement of electrons, the ultimate controls behind all body functions are all quite a mystery.

There is increasing scientific evidence that homeopathy works and a study of quantum mechanics has raised some interesting possible mechanisms through which homeopathic medicines may be able to exert their action. One needs to keep in mind that many essential trace elements and enzymes are present in very minute quantities and yet have profound effects on many systems within the body.

Secondly the action of many substances within the body may not always be due only to their chemical properties but due to their molecular structure and the molecular dynamics within the molecule. There are many unanswerable questions in science. This inability to explain does not constitute proof of non-action. In the meantime homeopaths and members of the public continue to use homeopathic remedies and continue to claim successful results.

The simple act of raising one's hand is an example of a small input having massive effects. The thought behind raising one's hand can't be measured and yet it sets into motion a whole range of physiological and anatomical effects. I believe there is a principle here, which perhaps also applies to the way in which homeopathic medicines may initiate a healing response.

The great initiators, explorers and researchers are those that don't accept the claims, theories, opinions and clever arguments of others but strike out in new directions. If something works, then all that is necessary is to find a theory or hypothesis that can explain those results and make them acceptable to others.

Natural Medicine (Naturopathy/Traditional systems):

This is the medicine of traditional people throughout the world. Natural suggests that it is a medicine that works with nature in a way that is natural. It is not surprising that traditional people should practise natural medicine. The modus operandi of these early people would obviously be developed from a study of nature, watching animals, the seasons, the movements of the planets and developing a sensitivity and an intrinsic 'feel' of the plant kingdom. They watched the flow of the seasons, the monthly cycle of women, the developmental stages of growth of plants, animals and humans, the natural healing of wounds and broken bones and recognised an intrinsic flow which seemed always to maintain a balance of function and maintenance of harmony within the body. It seemed appropriate therefore when the body was ill to assist this natural intrinsic movement towards harmony.

Rest, drinking of good clear water, fasting, and massage were certainly the earliest forms of supporting the ill person. This was natural healing and is still the most basic form of healing practised by most people all around the world. Herbs probably came later and were used also to support the natural healing processes. Music, singing, prayer were all natural attempts to influence healing and move the ill person from a state of disharmony towards health and harmony.

Basic to Natural Medicine was an understanding that order and disorder were flowing processes that followed intrinsic laws inherent in nature. If one disobeyed these laws, then ill health and disease were the natural outcome. The power of nature and its underlying laws were constantly moving and maintaining a balance of forces.

All that was required to move the ill person towards health again was an understanding of these laws and helping the system return to its previous harmony with itself and its environment. We will be dealing with these ideas much more fully in later chapters but already perhaps one can sense the power in the simplicity of the above state- ments.

This book is all about Natural Medicine in its very broadest sense. One must return back to these simple principles in order to make sense of the whole field of Complementary and Alternative Medicine and how this should be integrated into the medicine of today.

Naturopathic Medicine:

Practitioners of this medicine basically use the principles of Natural Medicine and techniques, which include water therapy, fasting and diets, herbs, massage, sauna, infrared radiation, etcetera.

Herbal Medicine (Phytotherapy):

Practitioners of this medicine specialise in the use of herbs and generally use other naturopathic approaches to stimulate healing which may include special diets, enemas, massage and exercise programmes.

Bioenergetic Medicine

This is a medicine of modern times and many practitioners believe that this is the direction medicine must move and will move as we develop more and more machines which can detect the energetic fields operating within the body. It seems that these fields can be seen and felt by many 'sensitives' who are able to make an energetic diagnosis of malfunction and also treat this energetic disturbance by the laying on of hands.

The early Chinese writings referred to energy flowing around the body along clearly indicated pathways. Recent attempts have been made to identify these pathways. It has been shown for example that acupuncture points have very low electrical resistance compared to other parts of the skin surface. Electronic machines have been developed based on this early work to detect changes in this electrical resistance and attempts have been made to quantify these measurements. A number of companies around the world now produce machines for detection and treatment based on these recordings.

Disease may be quantified by these practitioners as a disturbance of the energy dynamics and corrected by changing the energy readings towards normal. This research is still in its infancy but has an enormous potential in diagnosis of the potential towards disease patterns and the early energetic changes before there are any physical manifestations. A great deal of confusion arises because claims of disease are often made by practitioners using these machines when all that is recorded is energetic disturbances. Interpretation of the results requires experience and careful analysis based also on some understanding of variable flow of energy and attempts by the system to correct imbalances.

Acupuncture:

This is a technique of Traditional Chinese Medicine (TCM) and is really a part of a more holistic approach, which includes herbal medicine and massage. This system of medicine is thousands of years old and is once again having a resurgence of interest based on many scientific studies starting to show its efficacy in treating a number of pain conditions.

Ancient textbooks describe pathways of energy flowing along the body's surface with connections to the internal organs. Along the surface pathways are specific points which allow practitioners to change the dynamics of energy flow by inserting needles, using moxa (a technique of applying heat), and massage, low energy laser light or even injecting into these points. According to TCM any illness is due to an imbalance in the flow of energy, which manifests as symptoms and signs.

I have used acupuncture for about 25 years and I am convinced that it is one of the most useful of complementary approaches to healing. I have seen changes happen in front of me that have convinced me without any doubt that the conventional approach to treating disease is missing something very fundamental.

The butterfly effect of quantum mechanics has proven that small input can have massive effects and therefore weather prediction is so often unreliable. On a weekly basis I see my needles when applied to specific acupuncture points having profound effects that cannot be explained by any theory based on a conventional biochemical model of disease.

I know this is not a placebo response because using low energy lasers (to stimulate acupuncture points) that cause no sensation at all produce the same results as using needles. In addition to the use of needles and other techniques to stimulate acupuncture points, practitioners of TCM use herbs mixed according to ancient recipes that have been shown to have very deep acting and profound energy moving properties.

Ayurvedic Medicine:

This is the traditional medicine of India and is said to have originated even as far back as 40,000 years ago. The word literally means the 'Science of Life' and was collated in written form 5000 years ago. The basis of Ayurveda is the Theory of Tridosha. A dosha is a biological operating principle that functions throughout nature. The three doshas operating in human beings are Vata (wind), Pitta (fire) and Kapha (water). Each individual is a unique combination of these operating principles. Imbalance in the way these three doshas operate results in ill health, which can be corrected by bringing the system back into balance.

Ayurveda is a superb example of lifestyle management. It concentrates on diet (depending on the dosha), exercise (yoga), breathing techniques, detoxification, various rejuvenation therapies, sound therapy, language therapy and stress management. Herbal supplements are a valuable addition to these approaches.

There are also many other divisions of natural medicine such as aromatherapy, reflexology, Reiki, prayer, chiropractic and numerous massage and manipulative techniques. All these techniques and methods have a particular philosophical basis, which is generally based on ancient traditional principles or a more modern Holistic approach to natural medicine.

There are certainly common principles involved. The human being is an enormously complex anatomical, biochemical, energetic and informational system with deep and profound connections to other complex systems. The seemingly simple process of lifting one's hand up instigated by a thought, which has no idea about biochemistry, or anatomy is a miracle in itself.

There seems to be an intelligence operating within the biological system that can be called upon to assist in the healing process. I have no idea how to lift my hand up. The intelligence within the system seems to be able to respond to my wishes for the hand to go up. Any system of healing apart from the conventional model of medicine, which uses powerful drugs and surgery, is generally perfectly aware about the system's own innate intelligence and calls upon this intelligence to help in the healing process.

Nutritional Medicine:

Certain practitioners specialise in the use of nutritional substances which are substances derived from natural sources and usually include vitamins, minerals, amino acids, phyto-nutrients derived from herbs such as natural progesterone and phyto-estrogens, other hormone like substances derived from food sources such as DHEA, anti-oxidants, essential fatty acids such as the omega 3 and omega 6 fatty acids derived from fish oil and evening primrose oil respectively.

Definitions

These natural products are with increasing frequency and sophistication being combined in various formulas for specific effects and constitute one of the fastest growing markets all around the world. As indicated in chapter 2 processing does change these products and even the word natural becomes abused. The majority of vitamins sold in the market are synthetic and while they may act similarly to their natural counterparts are not 'natural' in the strict sense of the word.

The use of nutritional supplements in other than physiological doses, i.e. very high doses, is the approach of megavitamin therapy and orthomolecular medicine (see above). The value of nutritional medicine is definitely underrated by conventional doctors who have been sold the pharmacological package of using drugs to treat disease. Consider the following information:

- Low blood levels of vitamin E may be a better predictor of coronary heart disease than either elevated cholesterol levels or high blood pressure[1].

- Vitamin A deficiency in some countries is enormous and contributes for example to stunting and eye diseases.

- Vitamin supplementation is regarded as one of the most cost effective ways to reduce child mortality in Africa and other 3rd world countries.

- In the Linxian intervention trials carried out in China, small doses of vitamins and minerals led to statistically significant reduction in total mortality, reduction in cancer mortality, decreased incidence of cataracts and oesophageal cancer[2].

1   Gey,K; Puska,P et al (1991)'Inverse correlation between plasma vitamin E and mortality from ischemic heart disease in cross-cultural epidemiology' American journal of Clinical Nutrition 53(1Suppl) 326S-334S.

2   Blot WJ et al Nutritional intervention trials in Linxian,China: supplementation with specific vitamin/mineral combinations, cancer incidence, and disease-specific mortality in the general population. J Natl Cancer Inst.1993;85(18):1483-92

• 40% of the general population in America and 50% of all adolescents consume less than 2/3 of the RDA for vitamins and minerals largely due the high consumption of processed, fast and sugared foods. When one considers that magnesium is the activator for over 300 biochemical enzymes necessary for optimum metabolic wellbeing then one can understand that many of us are not functioning optimally[3].

The above information can be applied to many of the other nutrients i.e. deficiencies of vitamins, minerals and other nutrients exist right across the board. Few people probably have perfectly normal nutrients in optimum amounts. This means that many if not most human beings have less than optimum function due to nutritional deficiencies alone. It should be obvious that the better the body functions the better it can heal itself. Any deficiency will compromise the possibility of good function and healing and make the possibility of disease more likely.

Chiropractic:

This is perhaps the most well known of all the manipulative complementary approaches to wellness which includes Osteopathy, Rolfing, Shiatsu and many others. Like all the other professions chiropractic has undergone a plethora of innovations so that its boundaries have expanded and perhaps even blown apart. Many of the techniques no longer even look like the version originally formulated by Dr Daniel Palmer many years ago and practitioners now claim to treat a whole range of medical problems.

Chiropractors believe that mal-alignment of the spine, joints and muscles of the body lead to dysfunction of the body function and eventually disease. By correcting these misalignments, function can be returned to normal, pain is reduced and health returns. This is the basic principle of all the other manipulative therapies. It is significant that medical aids around the world are beginning to pay for chiropractic treatment. As indicated already and as will be emphasised over and

3   Lakshmanan F 'Magnesium intakes, balances and
     blood levels of adults consuming self-selected diets'
     The American journal of clinical nutrition
     40.Dec(1984) 1380-1389

over again throughout this book any method which increases function and improves health will decrease ill health.

The "New" Medicine:

Perhaps by the time this book is complete a new medicine will have already emerged. I don't believe it is quite here yet. It will certainly contain elements of all that has already presented itself both old and new but I believe we are in the middle of an evolutionary creative cycle.

When a new compound is formed the various elements which make up that compound suddenly combine in such a way that new properties emerge that no longer reflect the individual properties of the single elements. That is the difference between a mixture and a compound. I sense that this is happening to medicine today and that in the mixture which is occurring today we will slowly begin to see the making of a new medicine very different from its constituent parts. Practitioners will have to be very open minded and creative not to miss the signals being presented to them with the passage of time.

Other Therapies:

There are many other very powerful therapies available today. Some of these therapeutic approaches have become professions in their own right as they grow in status and develop clear indications and therapeutic skills. Such therapies include aromatherapy and reflexology while other therapies tend to be piggy backed and included into the armament of the various practitioners and therapists. These include colour therapy, radiesthesia, radionics and many others.

Chapter 6

We were in the far northern part of the famous Kruger National Park of South Africa and asked our guide to take us to the best known Traditional Healer in the area. There was a group of about twelve of us and we each wanted to experience a session with a 'Sangoma'[1].

The next day we were taken to a local village and each of us had a turn to be in the presence of this old African lady, perhaps 70 years old who sat on the mud floor and threw the bones on a skin mat in front of her.

The hut smelt of dry earth and dung and dry reed grass on the roof. The sangoma spoke some words and invited each of us in turn to sit down on the floor while she shook the bones in the bag they were in and then proceeded to spread them on the mat in front of her. Each bone, rock, and piece of wood represented some aspect of life and relationship to the world around, the way they lay, and the direction they pointed had a very clear meaning to the sangoma.

There was something quite sacred in the whole process. Perhaps it was just the setting, out in the African bush, surrounded by wild animals, sitting on a mud floor with this weathered old lady staring at the bones and finding meaning for each of us.

There were messages in the bones for each of us that immediately struck a note of the authenticity of the Sangoma and why she was highly respected in this area. As we drove back to our lodging place I could tell that each of us was lost in our own thoughts and how this unique experience had humbled us all. Out here in the African bush an elderly lady who knew nothing of our history could summon the voices of the ancestors through the fall of the bones and find meaning for us all on our journey in this life.

Experience and Experiment

A patient of mine asked me to speak to a certain sports medicine specialist about her medical condition. She was concerned about the long term prognosis and what it would do to her long term plans. During my conversation with this specialist I referred to the use

1   Traditional African shamanic healer

of low energy lasers which I use frequently in many sports injuries. His comment was that although he knew that many physiotherapists were using this device he had not seen any scientific studies to show that it was better than a placebo.

I tried to assure him that the laser really did work and that in my 35 years' experience I had seen very many remarkable results. He seemed uninterested in my experience and again pointed out that the scientific literature was unimpressive and that my experience was merely anecdotal.

I am always astonished at this attitude of many medical colleagues. Thirty five years' experience is no small matter. I trained 20 to 40 doctors every year in the use of the laser and they continue to confirm the remarkable benefits of such low energy lasers. All this is anecdotal of course and therefore no journal will publish such success stories.

I sometimes wonder what specialist this doctor would go to if he was ill, the specialist with 35 years experience or someone who knew all the latest literature but had very little experience. I have a text book in my possession in which there is a chapter on laser therapy written by a well known specialist who uses acupuncture needles to treat disease. In one chapter of the book the writer claims that there is no scientific proof that low energy lasers work. It beats me that the editors of the text book should ask a non believer who does not practise laser therapy to write a chapter on laser therapy.

This is an important issue because it has to do with the way of science and the nature of experience. Is science, with its double blinds and million dollar research programmes of more value than 10-20-30 years of experience? Is the young doctor full of enthusiasm and information better able to handle disease than the older doctor with the experience?

How valuable is experience compared to scientific methodology?

Information vs Experience

Medical journals will generally not print articles that deal with doctors' experiences but only articles which have followed the strict 'scientific' code of research which usually means double blind trials in reputable centres. This despite the fact that the FDA commissioner in America in 1978 testified to the Senate Health Subcommittee regarding the audits of 13 physicians who were doing drug trials for 48 major manufacturers and described the findings as horrible and inconceivable.

He told of reports on patients who did not exist, who never received the drug, who never gave consent to be tested, or who did not have the disease which the drug was supposed to treat or who were given dangerously high doses.

Diagnostic procedures in the USA amount to 40-50% of hospital charges and 10% of the total health care bill. A Harvard University hospital study compared the post mortem results during three ten year periods i.e. 1960-1970, 1970-1980 and 1980-1990. They found that the diagnostic errors were about the same in each ten year period despite the fact that the diagnostic procedures had increased in sophistication over these years.

A laboratory test study in Britain found that in only 2% of 174 emergency hospital admissions did tests performed result in change of treatment. The report stated that it is 'difficult to avoid the conclusion that these investigations were a waste of resources'[2].

These studies suggest that doctors still tend to respond to gut feeling and experience when making decisions even in critical situations. Perhaps they intuitively know that investigations are not all they are made out to be. What may seem as a very objective test is really a frozen section of a moment in time in a very dynamic system which has the ability to make very profound changes in fractions of seconds.

An X ray for example is a very limited view of the inside of the body. Although one uses a machine to take the X-Ray the interpretation is made by human beings and the machine itself has serious limitations as to what it can measure. It is often in the interpretation that scientific rationality begins to break down. Human beings do not function like machines.

It is not possible for them to be 100% objective because all data must enter into the brain and be interpreted. Cardiologists have been shown to vary by 60% in their assessment of coronary angiograms and surgeons when given case descriptions varied by 50% in their recommendations for surgery. Two years later the same surgeons changed their minds in 40% of the same cases.

Any interpretation is always conditioned by the person's culture, language, training, character, emotional state, physical health, etcetera.

2   Annals of clinical biochemistry 1980

Take into account also the limitations of any diagnostic machine which can only measure what it is made to measure and that is its inbuilt limitation.

Medical diagnostic devices give one view only

This must still be interpreted by a human being with varying degrees of training and experience.

Most people will experience at least one diagnostic error in their lifetime, sometimes with devastating consequences. This is not necessarily the fault of the doctor or the machines but due to the complexity of what it is one is trying to investigate. Conventional medicine chooses to focus on pathology because that is relatively easy to define and is less interested in disturbances of function which generally cannot be identified that easily until the condition is fairly serious and advanced.

The difficulty of translating from one language to another is because the meaning of the word in one language does not often have the exact equivalent in another language. If there is no exact equivalent word then the experience conveyed behind that word is also incorrectly interpreted. The language we use focuses our experience in particular ways. It also limits our experience. The Eskimos for example have numerous words to describe the objective nature of snow and their subjective experience of it. The English language is limited in its description of snow and therefore will also limit our ability to describe our experience.

Our interpretation of any phenomenon will therefore always be limited. Scientists understand this and therefore prefer to reduce all phenomenon to mathematics and statistics. It is at this level that science becomes impersonal, unam- biguous and objective.

The theory is great and certainly the numbers are objective and precise. The trouble is that they do not have anything to do with reality and the experience of that reality as we know it.

Reality is not a Mathematical Formula

Lorenz was a meteorologist. One evening he was playing around with some theoretical numbers on his computer. The numbers were to the 6th decimal place and he was working on theoretical weather patterns. With these numbers he obtained a particular weather forecast.

He decided to check the forecast again but because he was a little short of time he repeated the process but used the same numbers to the 3rd decimal place. When he returned a short time later to check the results he was astonished to discover that the predicted weather pattern with the numbers to the 3rd decimal place was very different to that with the numbers to the 6th decimal place.

'That these results were so far apart means that complex non-linear dynamic systems such as weather (and man) must be so incredibly sensitive that the smallest details can affect them.'

It is obvious now to most meteorologists that no matter how sophisticated the machines they use to predict the weather the accuracy of that prediction falls at an increasing rate the further forward they attempt to make the prediction. This is obvious to anyone who watches the forecasts on the television. What is astonishing is how very quickly that accuracy begins to fall. If this is true of weather then what about human beings?

No matter how sophisticated our machines, weather prediction will always be a combination of numbers generated, experience and guesswork.

Patients expect a great deal more from doctors than they can possibly deliver and will themselves confound predictions over and over again.

Is meteorology a science or an art? Do meteorologists arrive at their predictions based on science, gut feeling or experience. My old gardener was more often than not closer to the correct prediction about weather in our area than the newspaper or TV.

The Webster dictionary defines experience in the following ways:

• Direct observation of or participation in events: an encountering, undergoing, or living through things in general as they take place in the course of time.

• Knowledge, skill, or practise derived from direct observation or participation in events.

• Practical wisdom resulting from what one has encountered, undergone, or lived through.

• The sum total of the conscious events that make up an individual's life.

The key to experience is that it is an event of living systems. One does not expect a machine to have an experience nor of course does the mathematical formula have any experience of its own calculations. The experience has many qualities to it. It includes physical components, feeling, thinking, emotions, awareness, consciousness and an area of experience which falls outside consciousness which is referred to as intuition, subconscious, superconscious, or spiritual. This latter area is of immense importance and I will try to explore this area in a later chapter.

The Nature of Experience

It is interesting to compare education of children today and those of earlier times. My acupuncture teacher told me that his own teacher who is an old man now never had the formal training required in China today. His father allowed him to accompany him to the clinic as soon as he showed some interest. After some time he was allowed to hold the container with the acupuncture needles that his father used.

He did this for many years before his father allowed him to insert the needle into acupuncture points. There was very little formal teaching between the father and pupil. He was eventually given books to read and was allowed to ask questions which his father answered with great care.

From the very beginning the teaching was experiential. Today the emphasis in education is giving the student information. Although most medical education does contain a great deal of experience, this experience has no formal structure through which the student may enrich the process. Instead the overlay of science and emphasis on left brain approaches diminishes the value of the experience to the medical student. Science is measurement and has little to do with experience. As indicated above science does not want to hear about experience or one's personal viewpoint. All that is regarded as anecdotal and not science.

Anecdote[3]

Short narrative of an interesting, amusing, or curious incident often biographical and generally characterised by human interest.

3   Webster dictionary

Healthy Medicine

After 35 years in natural medicine I am a storehouse of anecdotes. The only ones interested in all this experience are my own colleagues who know the value of my experience but no medical conventional journal will publish this information despite the fact that I have been able to cure many conditions that their own specialists have failed to cure.

I wrote an article some time ago with the following title 'Acupuncture Revisited'. The article was returned with a request that I should leave out references to my experience and keep to the scientific facts. In other words it was okay to review articles on acupuncture but not to insert anecdotal information from my practise.

I telephoned the editor whom I knew personally and asked him why he was prepared to believe the research of doctors overseas whom he did not know but was not interested in my experience. The editor was sympathetic towards my viewpoint and decided to publish the article despite the reviewer's note that my article should not be published until I had removed these personal offending passages.

The ancient masters knew that experience requires special methods of teaching which are very different to the spoon feeding of information. Some of the requirements to refine the experience are the following:

- The student must be open minded and not stuck in a particular point of view i.e. no bias.

- There must be a great deal of self awareness. Too many of us are responding in a mechanical way to any stimulus without any awareness that our responses are mechanical.

- Emotions cloud my experience of this present moment. I should not be emotionally reactive in the presence of my patients. A state of inner peace would be most appropriate.

If I am angry then all I can experience is my own anger. Now this is okay if what I want to experience is anger but if I want to learn something about the patients and not just about myself then I need to be sure that my emotions are out of the way.

- My logical thinking mind should be as quiet as possible and even out of the way as much as possible during the consultation. This is the value of meditation which assists in learning to step back from thought. Thought is the buzz that constantly interferes with the silence of the moment. Just as the loud music in a nightclub interferes with a conversation so the constant rattle of our own thoughts interferes with what should be the refreshing signals of the experience between me and the patients. Our thoughts become the experience rather than the experience itself which is beyond thought.

• As thought and emotions become still a silence becomes apparent, the mind is no longer limited by any bias and like a deer standing with its ears alert, awareness is heightened. In that moment the experience moves outside the realm of self centredness into the transcendental.

This is of course the ideal and few of us perhaps reach this space but the closer we move towards this ideal not only is the experience more fulfilling but the response becomes more appropriate. Instead of reacting we can respond. Reaction come from self centredness. Response arises from some deep space within, in which self(ish) becomes Self(less).

Learning to Respond Rather than React Comes from Being in the Centre of the Experience

Scientists often point to the fact that many people are deluded by their own experience. We see things that don't exist and tend to overinflate or underrate the importance of a particular situation. This is no doubt true but then that is what experience is all about. The more experience one has the less one relies on the so called facts and the more one begins to trust oneself. Experience like every other human attribute improves with more experience.

A book appeared some years ago written by an eminent Professor of Surgery debunking all of natural medicine. The chapter on acupuncture was quite astonishing. Here was a doctor who had never practised acupuncture suggesting that acupuncture could not possibly work and was based on a philosophy which was archaic and primitive.

Statements like that are certainly not in the spirit of science which I believe should be open ended, creative and yes, experiential too. Experience is direct involvement. Mathematical formulas for all their power are only numbers on a piece of paper.

Statistics are also part of the numbers game but like weather prediction require human experience to add real value to their usage. At this moment I am sitting with a young lady of 22 years who is agonising over the decision whether to go for chemotherapy to treat her cancer or work to improve her health hoping that this will be able to control the cancer. The stakes are high.

She has an unusual and aggressive form of cancer. The oncologists have little experience in this form of cancer and are unable to hazard a prediction about the outcome of the treatment. The treatment itself is life threatening and she will lose all her hair. They have given her the statistics but there is no way of knowing what her fate is until it has happened. My experience is worth little as I have never seen a case like this before. What does the young lady do? I suggest she follow her heart and be true to her inner voice.

Life in the beginning and the end will always remain a game of chance. Will one's choices be made on the numbers game or does one choose a path with a heart which reaches into the very essence of oneself. It seems to me that very often one makes ones choices based on apparent logic and accumulation of facts because it somehow seems safer and at least there is someone else to blame if it does not succeed.

Experience is a slow teacher and turns us more often than not to a deeper knowing , a gut feeling , some deep stirring of truth, a light that needs to be followed into the unknown. Logic and statistics creates the illusion that the future is known and predictable and therefore there seems some safety in the process.

As weather prediction indicates, this sense of safety in the future is an illusion and cannot be trusted anymore perhaps than our own experience. Yet as experience in listening to one's heart grows more open to outcomes, there begins to emerge a truth which transcends time and space and moves us towards appropriate actions which synchronise with the present moment. This movement is often referred to as intuition.

Responding to the Heart or to the Head, Intuition or Logic?

It may seem strange to say that science is always old and experience always new but the truth is that science is always based on so called facts and facts, by their very nature must be measurable, relatively stable and move in a predictable way and belong to the past.

If the objects of measurement were not stable and were unpredictable then the science of these objects would indeed be very difficult. The data collection process is always of the past and may not be relevant in a world of change and has little to say about the individual patient sitting in front of the doctor.

We can return now to the weather and biological systems. They do not conform to the material objects that science likes to deal with. They are most difficult to hold down and will not follow any predictable path so that weather prediction is a guessing game based on numbers. Science can only deal with these living systems by using statistics which are based on past measurements.

Experience on the other hand is a very different process. Although memory is involved this memory is very different to that stored in a computer because it is not numbers but a living experience of the past events and takes the present conditions into account, searching within for correspondences and associations and using intuition which transcends time and space.

Through this very human process an answer arises that is most appropriate for the situation as it is at that moment. This is still an imperfect process because we are dealing with complexity and an insurmountable amount of unknown factors. Nevertheless science without experience loses its richness and even relevance for the patient who is ill.

Science Deals with the Past, Experience Brings the Present Moment into Context

Experience teachers one that each person is unique and cannot be dealt with as a statistic. Human beings are inconsistent in their responses and this applies not only to their emotional responses but even to the way they respond to physical agents. Dust may cause a hay fever attack in one person, a blocked nose in another, an asthmatic attack in a third and a cough in a fourth person.

Even in the same individual the nature of the response to dust will often have characteristics which are different to the previous attack. The left nostril may be blocked rather than the right and the eyes may be more itchy than on the previous occasion.

Experience understands these paradoxes and the mystery of life and seeks to find an appropriate response and meaning in this particular time frame. Experiment on the other hand gives us numbers, formulas and standard protocols of management. Experience when used wisely always has the advantage because it never excludes the results of experiments but recognizes it as one of the tools used to investigate the now. Those that rely on experiment tend to deny their own innate God given faculties and look to sources outside themselves for answers.

Practitioners of Natural Medicine are often asked about the science in what they are doing. The truth is that they are less interested in the science and more interested in the experience. In order to raise the experience to its highest level requires an enormous amount of skill and self evaluation.

If experience is to become meaningful in one's life and practice there is a need for constant self evaluation to get rid of self or selfishness, to have a degree of inner peace and compassion for the other, to be attentive and have a listening ear as described above. It is in this way that one's experience develops into a creative force which is able to respond to each challenge with an appropriateness that cannot be matched by science and its numbers.

Chapter 7

Many clients are intrigued by their first visit to my rooms. Firstly there is the half kilometre drive along a farm gravel road which can be quite hectic in winter and then sitting in the waiting room looking out onto a garden of trees and shrubs and birds darting around.

A patient once said to me that whenever she was ill she would first drive past my place and if she was not better after that she would then make an appointment. Just the drive was enough to stimulate healing.

I often wonder why it is that some patients never improve no matter what treatment they follow and then suddenly for the most inexplicable reason all their symptoms disappear and life carries on. What really is the role of doctors and healers in this process?

Are doctors healers, educators or dispensers of medicines. Are doctors magicians, alchemists or manipulators of energy. The attitude they take will often define the system of medicine they follow but how important is it to the sick person?

Two Medicines, Two Systems

I have studied two systems of medicine, which are so different that it seems at times not possible to integrate them. There is a good reason for this difference and this has been reviewed in the chapters on the history of Western medicine and Natural medicine.

The system of natural medicine that I am familiar with is Traditional Chinese Medicine (TCM). The philosophy of TCM is often dismissed by Western doctors as archaic and not scientific. This is not a helpful attitude to take as it denies that person the enormous learning that is possible with a system of medicine that has not only survived more than two thousand years but is still practised today and even used in Chinese Traditional Hospitals to treat people with serious conditions.

I have been using acupuncture for more than 35 years and have too much respect for this very ancient form of treatment to feel that I can dismiss the philosophy, which supports the treatment process. Nevertheless other medical doctors have managed to separate the philosophy and practice in what they call 'Medical Acupuncture'.

With time however, I have begun to understand the nature of this difference between different systems of medicine and would like to share with you some of these insights which will help to clarify why it is that there are so many different systems of healing and how each can still claim to heal disease.

As my interest in natural medicines grew I started to experiment with various products that came to my attention. I was soon astonished to discover that when given for the right indications there were usually very clear and observable results.

Homeopathy with its very strange formulations in particular surprised me; that minute doses of medicines could obtain results even in very serious and obviously physical diseases. As a medical student I was already familiar with herbal medicine. The very early medicines were in fact the powerful herbs such as digitalis used for heart failure, colchicine used for gout, belladonna used as an antispasmodic and rewolfia used for hypertension.

Herbalists interestingly enough today seldom use these herbs because they are regarded as poisonous and could lead to litigation problems for them. Doctors of conventional medicine have no problem on the other hand using drugs with serious side effects. Most drugs have potentially serious side effects but doctors understand that this comes with the package.

Doctors believe that the benefits of using drugs are worth the risks.

I was soon to discover however that in using natural products, even though they are much less powerful than drugs and therefore don't have major toxic effects, that real healing benefits were still possible. The strong poisonous herbs acted much more like drugs while the apparently weaker herbs had a much more sustained and deeper healing benefit on the physiological processes within the body. It seemed that they supported health rather than treated the disease and therefore did not need to be powerful.

As the years went by I began to introduce nutritional substances such as the vitamins and minerals, trace elements, natural bio-identical hormones, enzymes, other food supplements, homotoxiological remedies, diet therapy, energy medicine, flower essences, gemmotherapy and many others. Each had their particular place and indications.

At first my enthusiasm knew no boundaries but slowly and with increasing speed I soon became quite confused trying to follow each philosophy and mixing the various remedies in the treatment of the many patients with chronic disease that increasingly came to see me. Everything worked if the indications were right and yet all the philosophies seemed to be different and certainly there was an enormous difference between homeopathy, herbal medicine, acupuncture and psychotherapy.

So what was going on? Were there common principles involved despite what appeared to be very different philosophies and the use of different products and techniques? It seems that the human mind has no end to inventiveness. One God it seems but many religions and many interpretations. Each person believing that their way is the only right way. Perhaps we need to examine also if there are common principles in religious beliefs. This might resolve much of the conflict present in the world today.

The same problem exists in medicine where the conventional medical paradigm believes that it is on a high moral and scientific ground and most other forms of healing are not scientific and therefore should not be considered for the treatment of ill health. The thinking is that if healthy individuals want to take these nutritional products then that's okay. Sick individuals should however only be treated by conventional doctors using drugs and surgery when appropriate.

Many Different Therapies which all seem to have Therapeutic Effects in the Same Conditions

Experience and personal preferences in time created a personalised philosophy and approach to treatment. There are principles which are common, and we will deal with this in later chapters. I wish however in this chapter to clarify the difference between Western medicine and TCM so that we can move towards an understanding of how an integration of all these methodologies may be possible.

Let us consider for the moment a computer. A mechanical engineer, an electrical engineer, and a programmer would all have a different view of the computer. For the mechanical engineer the structure would be important, for the electrical engineer the electrical connections and the flow of electricity in the computer would be of special interest and for the programmer only the informational systems would be of interest. Each specialist would have a different view of the computer and would have a different language and approach to dealing with colleagues.

Something similar has happened in dealing with human beings and their ill health. This has arisen from the different viewpoint that groups of scientists have taken, based on the particular window through which each group has looked out onto the scene as observed from their own particular window. I live in a valley surrounded by mountains and it always fascinated me that from each mountaintop the valley looked completely different. The same valley, but different views. The same computer with many different professionals accessing it from different windows of interest. The same human being, but different systems of medicine.

Traditional Chinese doctors knew that the body had physical organs, tissues, muscles, etc., but they chose to view the human being from a perspective that supported their philosophy and used a window of perception that modern medical doctors regard as archaic. Let us for a moment look through each window in turn and see what it is that makes each system so different.

We have already alluded to the Western medical model, which has a window built by the Cartesian/Newtonian Company of engineers. The window is structured in such a way that from every viewpoint the objects in the world seem to be constructed from basic building blocks much like clay bricks are used to build a house. Whether the object is a human being or a building, an animal or a lamppost, all the objects living or dead, animate or inanimate appear to be made up of separate pieces held together in clearly defined ways.

A building is made of bricks held together by cement, a machine is made of strips of metal welded or screwed together and a human being is made up of cells linked together by nerves, blood vessels and intercellular tissue.

According to this approach human beings like the building or machine can be separated into parts and each part examined separately. Parts can be replaced or repaired or even removed entirely. If the person is ill then one can search through the body looking for the part that is disturbed or broken.

Enormous efforts are made to investigate the body with more and more sophisticated machines, chemical analysis of the blood, biopsy of tissues and surgery. Cameras and scopes are pushed into the body, X-rays, sonars and MRIs scan the body, looking for abnormalities. If nothing can be found, then either the problem is considered psychological, too small to be identified yet, or the tests are considered inadequate and other tests are performed or new tests invented based on the same model.

The Human Being is a Machine made up of Parts, which can be removed and replaced when Necessary.

When no pathology can be found and the tests come back normal then doctors will generally suggest a repeat visit in a few weeks time, do more tests and trials of various medications hoping that the condition will either clear up or become obvious over time.

This is exactly what happened to a 60 year old man who came to see me with regular (weekly) episodes of deafness on one side lasting hours and then hearing returning to normal. The ENT doctor could find nothing wrong and sent him home without any drugs and told him to return if the condition kept recurring which it did.

An MRI was ordered and the report came back normal. He realised that the ENT doctor was a bit stuck and came to see me. I prescribed some nutritional medicines with trace minerals, omega 3 and vitamin D and three weeks later his attacks had disappeared.

The specialist could not find any pathology and therefore could only send him home without any medicine as he did not know what the problem was and wait for the condition to express itself further. All I did was to support health and the body's own innate intelligence did the repair work. Neither the specialist nor I had a diagnosis but as an Integrative doctor I knew how to improve function.

Here are some interesting quotes by specialists in 'reductionistic' scientific medicine.

'In Science man is a machine for if he is not, then he is nothing at all.'[1]

'One of the acid tests of understanding an object is the ability to put it together from its component parts. Ultimately molecular biologists

---

1   Joseph Needham(1928)

will attempt to subject their understanding of cell structure and function to this sort of test, by trying to synthesise, a cell.'[2]

As this viewpoint of the body as a machine developed and became more entrenched and complex, specialists were required to examine the parts that were separated from the whole. Some general practitioners became specialists and surgeons also began specialising in body parts. An army of support teams followed and research became more and more specialised and narrow down to the field that the specialist was particularly interested in. The human being was often left out of the picture. Who needed the human being when one was examining the liver for example?

Modern medicine became more and more concerned with treating the diseased part and less concerned with the person who was ill. The person, in a certain sense, did not exist for science. He could not be measured. What could be measured was sodium, potassium, cholesterol and many other elements, the blood could be seen under the microscope and electron microscopy could even identify the cells and the intracellular components.

But the Human Being, from a Scientific Point of View, was Nowhere to be seen.

Electrons, protons and other particles were discovered as science penetrated further and further into the small and smaller components of the body parts and the person seem to vanish further away with each deeper level of penetration.

This approach to the investigation of biological systems and human beings in particular, inevitably let to some obvious conclusions. As scientists penetrated deeper into the system and separated the whole into more and more parts, the human element seemed to disappear.

Consciousness, mind, soul and spirit were not there. Even emotions and thought, love and compassion, willpower and awareness could not be measured directly. The logical conclusion from this kind of research was that these qualities were not real but an epiphenomenon i.e. a secondary factor arising out of the workings of matter. Sodium and potassium and all the parts of the body had somehow over time learnt to think and feel.

2   American textbook of Biology.

It was felt that the human component was like a cloud excreted or emitted by the physical components much like speech may be regarded as the result of the vocal cords moving in a certain way as air passes through. The human component cannot be measured. Try sending blood away to the laboratory and requesting information about the person rather than the body parts. Even though doctors often refer to depression as a chemical problem there is no diagnostic test for this condition. Nor is there a diagnostic test for happiness or sadness, for joy or anger, for inner peace or inner emotional chaos.

All these latter conditions are more easily identified by other human beings than by machines or physical tests.

Matter is basic, the "Human Being" is Secondary and a Later Development on the Evolutionary Scale.

The window of TCM gives us a very different view of the human being. Understandably so because the glass spanning the window is not divided into squares, which give the brick like effect of the modern Western approach, but is instead in a fluid state so that all objects seem to be made up of flowing materials that have no clearly defined borders, but appear to merge into and out of centres of activity; much like sea water rolls in eddies and whirlpools onto the beach and then flows back again. If one watches very carefully it almost seems as if there are underlying controls within the flowing processes guiding the movement of flow. What one sees appears secondary to an underlying energetic shift.

This viewpoint is almost the exact opposite of the one above. Firstly everything flows and is in a constant process of change. Secondly the more obvious physical states which can be seen and measured are secondary to the underlying energetic states which hold the flowing physical characteristics in shape and control. There even seem to be deeper and more subtle levels of energy. This is discussed in later chapters especially the chapter on anatomy.

The 'Human Being' is made up of Flowing Systems

One could ask of course, which is the reality? The brick-like human being or the flowing-system human being. It seems that the window of perception is creating the 'illusion' or 'reality' of the object human being. Which is the correct interpretation? Are human beings a collection of cells or are human beings a flowing system?

Looking out through the one window gives one view and looking out through the other window gives another view. Wearing blue glasses will make the world seem blue and red glasses will make the world appear red. Is the world red or blue? Does it all depend on the window one looks through?

One could say therefore that the world has no fixed reality, that it is the window of perception, which sets the tone for the view one has. It is important to understand this. It will help us all to overcome conflict of interests and perhaps also give us an interest in another person's point of view, which may give some insight into a fuller picture of reality.

What does become clear from the above discussion is that it is not either-or but rather and-and. Each window is another viewpoint only and each adds to the total picture. Each mountaintop I climb around my valley provides me with a fuller picture of the valley. Each system of medicine similarly can only enrich the limited viewpoint which one system has of the total human being.

This conflict around the nature of reality is not new to scientists. The study of light for example has found that light may be a particle or wave depending on the way we decide to measure it. Strangely, scientists can't measure both properties at the same time. Light is either particle or wave when measured. It is as if conventional medical scientists choose to see the human being as particle only while the TCM practitioner recognises the wave properties of human beings. Both are true and yet give a different perception of the same object being examined.

Reality is Only a Window of Perception

The TCM practitioners saw flowing systems within the human body. These flowing systems had areas of activity, which seemed to control the way in which the activity was directed and the pattern it shaped itself into. In health these flowing systems moved in a harmonious way and filled all areas of the body with a uniform and vibrant activity.

In disease there were areas of stagnation, deficiency or excess. When this occurred then symptoms and signs appeared and if this disturbed activity went on long enough then a crystallization or disruption of the physical matter would occur. In other words there was first a disturbance of the dynamics of flow, which eventually resulted in an actual appearance of disease in the physical body.

According to TCM understanding the disturbance of flow was at the level of energy. The TCM practitioners were not referring to the flow of blood or fluid or chemicals, but to a more subtle flow of energy. This energy was the ground substance upon which chemistry and anatomy rested and was directed.

Disturbances to Flow resulted in Disharmony and Disease

Imagine a large magnet covered by a thin cardboard sheet upon which are placed iron filings. The iron filings will take the shape of the magnetic field. If the field is changed, then the iron filings will change position to conform to the field. In a similar way the flow of energy or Qi was the ground substance as it were of the material body. The physical shape and substance took its cue from the underlying flow of energy, just as the iron filings moved to the underlying magnetic field.

In TCM, 'liver', for example, is not an organ, but an energetic blueprint, which includes the energetic image of liver organ plus a range of other energetic functions. All these functions are designated as the 'liver orb' and have influences all around the body. Thus disturbances in this energy field could affect the liver function, but may also express itself in the eyes or emotions, depending where these energetic disturbances were focused in the physical body.

I was always fascinated by this explanation because it gave me an answer to two riddles that have always puzzled me i.e. what and where are the controls in the body and how to fit in emotions, mind and spirit. The latter don't fit very comfortably into the Western medical model and tends to be regarded as an epi-phenomenon or appendage of the physical body.

In the TCM model however these aspects of a human being can be arranged in a clearly defined and creative way. What are the controls which prevent a simple cut from ending up as a mass of confused tissue cells rather than a paper-thin scar and each cell in near perfect arrangement to the surrounding tissue.

Clearly one answer is that behind the physical presence of cells and organs is an energetic field similar in its control function to a magnetic field. That is the way TCM understands the dynamics of the control system. We will discuss these two riddles in more detail in later chapters.

As indicated, the window of perception of the Western medical model created a reality in which the human being was made up of parts while the TCM window of perception created a reality in which the human being was made up of flowing energy. There is a similar conflict of interest between the old Newtonian physics and modern quantum physics.

Newtonian physics deals with macro-molecules, with the billiard balls moving across the table while quantum physics deals with the subatomic world, with electrons and protons and the energies which surround them. It is of interest that at one time it was felt that these two worlds, the macro-molecular world and the subatomic world had little in common.

It was felt that they could be studied totally separately as if there was an invisible wall between them. In recent times this wall is becoming thinner and thinner and many scientists now dare to question this separation and are suggesting that the one may influence the other.

Is the Human Being made up of Parts or Flowing Systems?

As already indicated light is both particle and wave and yet both cannot be measured at the same time. This is a very interesting dilemma for scientists.

It all depends it seems on the observer and the way in which he attempts to measure light. Similarly a human being could be both parts and flowing systems. It all depends as indicated above which window one looks through or which tools one uses to assess him or her. Under the microscope nothing flows and only interesting objects are seen.

There is a great need for a much fuller and whole view of people. Modern medical science, which is still very much stuck in the Newtonian Cartesian viewpoint, has reduced us all to bits and pieces of body stuck together. While emotions, mind and spirit may be accepted by individual doctors, these qualities as indicated have a very uncomfortable place in the anatomy of humans for the simple reason that none of these qualities can be measured. There is no large picture, no spiritual influence, no grand design, no magic or mystery. A physical body, which in time grows old and dies only to disintegrate back into the earth out of which its substance came.

The TCM view shows us another picture and this view has also been elaborated in modern times both by quantum scientists and systemic scientists. These scientists have developed modern counterparts to many of the ancient philosophies and ideas, moving away from isolated parts towards the idea of flowing systems, energy, informational transfer, dynamic and creative responses to small input and communication at a distance. These ideas have developed outside TCM and without knowledge of Traditional systems of understanding. The systems model of human beings is important to an understanding of Natural medicine and this will therefore be elaborated in the chapter on systems.

While I have used the TCM model in the chapter and compared it to the conventional medical viewpoint, any one of the other traditional systems of healing could be equally chosen. They have all developed an understanding of the human being as a flowing system connected to the whole with energy and informational transfer within the system.

In other chapters we will elaborate further into the significance of this difference because it will highlight major differences in approach to diagnosis, management and treatment.

Chapter 8

It has been a very dry summer and as I watch the rain I am very much aware of how the thirsty earth and plants have been waiting for this moment.

I like to think about the fact that trees give off oxygen, that my lungs absorb the oxygen and breathe out the carbon dioxide that the trees absorb. In this way there is a constant cycle of oxygen and carbon dioxide moving between my lungs and the trees. My body and the trees are linked together in a most profound relationship. My survival is dependent on them and while the trees are outside my body and therefore apart from me, they are at the same time part of the in-breath / out-breath system which makes up my respiratory system.

Perhaps my skin also does not separate me from the environment, but joins me to it. What about consciousness and mind? Am I also connected to the flow of consciousness that joins all of us together?

Properties of Biological Systems

The great shock of the 20th century science has been that systems cannot be understood by analysis. The properties of the parts are not intrinsic properties, but can be understood only within the context of the larger whole. Thus the relationship between the parts and the whole has been reversed. In the systems approach, the properties of the parts can be understood only from the organisation of the whole. Accordingly, the systems' thinking does not concentrate on basic building blocks but rather on basic principles of organisation.'[1]

The 'shock' of this information may be so great that most scientists are still in denial. Living things are not made up of parts but are functioning systems in which parts do not really exist. One could say that a system flows and is in a constant process of change so that nothing is really fixed. While thinking of building blocks is a good idea

1   Fritjof Capra 'The Web of Life'

for building a house or other structure this is not appropriate for living systems.

Life lives and this living quality manifests as metabolic processes, growth, reproduction and adaptation to the environment. This is not the nature of a building which is in a constant state of deterioration. So while it is appropriate at times to think of the liver, kidney, head, arms, blood etc. these are only the visible anatomical side of the body and are useful descriptions for a surgeon or pathologist.

There is however also the functional process side where flowing and changing is the order of the day and where to think of parts is not appropriate. Just as light can be thought of as having both particle and wave properties so the body can be thought of as having parts and process properties. To a surgeon the part properties are more important and to think of the body as similar to a building is more useful and appropriate.

When one considers ill health however it is sometimes more useful to think of the flowing processes and what interferes with flow. We should not wait until something breaks down and becomes 'visible' before doing something active. At this point only surgery or symptomatic treatment may be possible.

Before a motor breaks down it may be out of tune for a long period of time. This 'out of tunement' manifests as a change in function which is generally picked up by the driver as some very subtle changes in the way the car is operating. It may even manifest as an almost subliminal uneasiness one has when driving the car. This is similar to the uneasiness one has about something just surfacing in consciousness around the way our own bodies are operating.

With time it becomes clear that something is really wrong with the motor car or with our bodies and a second opinion becomes necessary. If nothing is done then eventually the motor car or the body breaks down and the broken part needs to be replaced in the motor car or surgery becomes necessary in the body.

It is this shift from flow to breakdown which characterizes the difference between the conventional medical viewpoint and a more systemic viewpoint.

What is a system?

Systems are integrated wholes whose properties cannot be reduced to those of smaller parts unlike machines which are made up of interlinking parts joined together.

Tease parts open to examine function and flow.

Break a system up and discover parts only, which do not flow.

The fascination of science in its early days was in breaking things apart to try and identify 'what was inside'. It seemed that by doing this, one would eventually come to the simplest building block out of which all things were created. The whole evolutionary process assumed that from these very simple elementary particles life was eventually created and while stones and rocks do not exhibit life as we understand it, biological systems have properties of living systems which are characteristically flowing in nature. This is very different to the way a building or other physical object increases in size and complexity.

So in this chapter we are going to look at properties of living systems. It's a good idea while reading through what follows that one keeps in mind the difference between these properties and what one would expect from a building. Keep in mind however that we are referring to the construction and structure of the building because even a building, to make it work and 'function', still requires the flow of information from one part of the building to another, so that even in a building one can recognize the difference between structure and flow.

What flows is more subtle and invisible. The electrical cables can be seen but not the electricity or the information. The telephone is seen but not the voice carried along the wires. The human body is seen but not the emotions or thoughts of the person. Flow is everywhere but generally invisible.

Structure vs Flow

Part vs Process

Particle vs Wave

Brain vs Mind / Consciousness

Properties of Biological Systems

1: Multi-Dimensional

Biological systems do not function in one dimension only but as indicated in other chapters have many different levels; anatomical and mechanical, biochemical, energetic, mind and consciousness, spirit and soul.

'Reality is a rich tapestry of interwoven levels, reaching from matter to body to mind to soul to spirit. Each senior level 'envelops' or 'enfolds' its junior dimensions – a series of nests within nests of being – so that every thing and events in the world are interwoven by spirit, by God, by Goddess, by Tao, by Brahman, by the Absolute itself.'[2]

According to Wilber each level of reality has a branch of knowledge associated with it so that physicists for example would study the physical body, psychology and philosophy addresses the mind, Theology studies the relationship to God, Mysticism studies the formless Godhead or pure emptiness and the nature of spirit.

The science of human beings and ill health tends to deal only with part of the whole, that part which can be measured relatively easily and in this way we tend to gain a much distorted view of human beings.

Human Beings are Multidimensional. We are not bodies only but matter-energy-informational beings.

The Cause of Ill Health may not only be at One Level but on Other Levels / dimensions as well.

2: Highly Complex

Biological systems are highly complex. So complex in fact that scientists are beginning to realise that they may not ever understand fully the nature of life or how it is co-coordinated and functions. Uncertainty is everywhere and weather prediction for example may never become much more accurate than it is today. In these highly complex systems a very small input may have very deep and profound effects which may be catastrophic or move the system into a higher level of functioning.

2   Ken Wilber, The Marriage of Sense and Soul (Random House)

This is known as the 'butterfly' effect. A butterfly flapping its wings in New York can cause a storm in San Francisco. Some cosmologists have been so impressed with this sensitivity of systems and how small input can have massive effects that they have speculated that there must be some intelligence operating and controlling because otherwise the universe would not have developed in such a uniquely co-coordinated and harmonious way. Even God as a reality has become a meaningful answer for many of these scientists.

The enormous complexity and sensitivity of biological systems should also make us very cautious in interfering with this system. Genetic modification is an example of this haphazard interference where not nearly enough is known to allow this introduction into our food supply without a great deal more research.

The complexity of living systems should make us very wary of thinking that we really know what is going on. On the other hand there does seem to be an underlying intelligence at work. Perhaps we can learn to work with this intelligence?

3: Biological Systems are Open Systems

One of the most important properties of biological systems is that they do not function in isolation. This is one of the most fundamental concepts of the new science and systems thinking.

Cells in the body communicate with other cells, glands communicate with other glands, brain communicates with body parts via nerve processes, the immune systems receives and sends information throughout the flowing systems of the body. There is also a profound communication system with the world around on a physical, emotional, mental and spiritual level.

Sounds, smells and colour have a whole range of influences. We receive and emit them all. Energy in the form of electromagnetic signals moves through us and we in turn send out electromagnetic messages and information. The recordings of the ECG i.e. the electrocardiogram reading of the heart can be taken three feet away from the body with very sensitive instruments. What does this say about heart to heart conversations?

While the electromagnetic spectrum may include the full range of signals recognised by scientists there are probably other ways that information may be transferred. This would explain the power of prayer, various other healing modalities, mental telepathy and how animals read information such as when a flock of birds twist and turn together or a quarter mile long shoal of fish will often respond together when a predator approaches. These all appear to be more subtle energies which may be outside the conventional electromagnetic spectrum as we know it.

So we are clearly not closed systems independent of outside influences. Perhaps if we recognised just how interconnected we were to the world around us, and of course to other human beings, we would deal much more kindly and sympathetically to others and to the plant and animal kingdom, with a deepening respect for life around us.

The skin does not separate us from our environment but joins us to it. Our lungs are open to the outside and breathes in molecules of air that have been emitted by trees and other human beings and animals. Those molecules are incorporated into the structure of our bodies. Our bodies are recycling material constantly, in the air, from the water and food we take in. If information is attached to these molecules then we recycle both material substance and information that has been elsewhere and we in turn pass material plus information onwards.

4: Non-linear

This is a difficult concept to get our heads around so be patient with yourself and read up as much as you can on this interesting and exciting topic because it will have a very deep and profound effect on you if you can fully integrate these ideas into your reality.

In the real world there are very few Cause - - - > Effect phenomena. Everything is affected by everything else.

'Thou can'st not stir a flower
without disturbing a star.'[3]

Newtonian science is often referred to as the billiard ball science. A billiard ball hitting another billiard ball will move in a particular direction based on speed, weight and trajectory which can be easily calculated if one knows all the parameters.

Biological systems are however not billiard balls. They are complex, multidimensional and open systems. So much is happening in any moment of time that it becomes impossible to measure all these parameters. The classic example is the weather. Despite all our measurements, predictions are just that, a good guess for tomorrow but the chances of being right begin to fall dramatically the further in the future we try and predict the weather.

3   Francis Thompson

Why this is so and what does it mean for healers and those that are ill?

This very moment referred to as the 'NOW' is not the end point of an event in the past but the fullness of the present. By this I mean everything known and unknown, past present and even the future comes together in this moment of time. What we are conscious of is only a small part of this moment. What can be measured is only a small part of this now.

What science can measure is only what it can measure and that is its limitation.

Non linear dynamics recognizes the difficulties of trying to link events. Behind the backdrop of what can be known is the 'great mystery', the 'unknown', the quantum potential and is a black hole of possibly infinite potentials.

It is the recognition that we are always dealing with unknown factors and that these unknown factors may be more important than the known factors that makes the NOW so special and unique and this is why exact prediction is practically and theoretically impossible. It should be obvious that if we don't know the unknown and that this has an influence on the known then not only is future prediction impossible but also trying to trace backwards to the cause will be equally impossible.

This moment is unique and will never be repeated in exactly the same way again.

This moment is also not just the end point of some cause in the past.

Each person's illness is unique in its own right and the diagnostic label should not fool us into thinking that we now understand what is going on or that everyone else with the same label has the same problem.

5: Creativity

Creativity accounts for the beauty, surprise and wonder found in nature.

It is a fundamental property of living systems that they are able to adapt and change.

This property is important and is used by doctors of integrated medicine to nudge living systems to find new ways to heal when there are obstructions to flow that cannot be changed.

The creativity of living systems is quite extra-ordinary and seems to be present right down to the smallest living things, such as viruses which are able to adapt and change to diverse circumstances. Drug resistance and new outbreaks of infectious disease attest to this remarkable creativity. Similar creativity can be seen in the way the immune system is able to handle the vastly increased amounts of new chemicals thrown at it.

If one considers the intelligence with which the human system is able to deal with so much complexity and the creative processes which constantly appear, then one must be left with a sense of awe that this intelligence could also be aware of itself and know what is going on. Now that thought could take us to some very interesting conclusions.

'All in all, the creativity of the living world is only a problem if we insist in trying to reconcile it with the paradigm of science.'[4]

It is not our remedies that are creative, but the way the body is able to use the remedies and approaches with which we try to heal. This creativity also suggests that presence of intelligence able to respond to the multiple pressures all around.

6: Purposeful / Goal Seeking

Living systems function in a purposeful way. They procreate, seek food and shelter, care for their young, avoid danger and prepare to die. Human beings may have additional goals such as pushing themselves to the edge of possibilities, wanting to be rich for all kinds of different reasons and spiritual goals.

Survival goals may seem easy to understand and certainly they must be connected into the genetic memory but exactly how this memory is imprinted and what triggers and directs this process has not been clearly elucidated. Spiritual goals are another matter.

4   The Way, an Ecological World View, Edward
     Goldsmith 1992

There are physical goals directed towards survival, emotional goals directed towards pleasure and various spiritual goals such as service, self enhancement etc.

What happens when these goals move in different directions? Could this contribute to ill health?

7: Living systems are Dynamic

A rock is static. Living systems on the other hand are constantly flowing, turning and twisting, contracting and relaxing, breathing in and breathing out, digesting and excreting. Even if the mind is completely still, the 'life' in the system is in constant motion. Like a Mexican wave in a stadium full of fans, wave after wave of activity streams through the human body system.

Even at night there is this constant streaming going on so that from going to bed tired and even exhausted, one wakes up feeling refreshed and alert. The body has done its work done its work of re-tuning the system and one is ready for the day.

The changing weather patterns and temperature of the day all require that adjustments are made in the body. With each emotion streaming through the body and directions from the mind to move and do, all happening very often at the same time the amount of activity would require a few buildings filled with computers to co-ordinate.

Where are the controls for all this activity?

There was a time when doctors would refer to the 'life force' and perhaps even today modern doctors talk about 'life flowing out of the body' or of someone having a 'weak life force' but such ideas of a life force are discredited by modern scientists. Life to a medical scientist has to do with the flow of biochemistry and this flow is co-coordinated by hormones, neurotransmitters, immunomodulators and there is no deeper organising force or energy.

Traditional systems of healing instead suggested that the life force was the organising and controlling 'energy' pulsing through the body and maintaining the balance of forces. While conventional science may not be able to measure such energy , the idea of a deeper controlling energy field should not be discarded in the face of complexity and how this is co-ordinated and managed.

There is more to a living body than just biochemistry.

The eyes tell us another story. They sparkle or are dull, they are humorous or warm, they are dark and mysterious or open and loving. The non measurable components are the qualitative aspects of that life force.

8: Maintenance of Balance and Harmony - Homeostasis

Tabers medical dictionary defines homeostasis as a state of equilibrium of the internal environment of the body that is maintained by dynamic processes of feedback and regulation. Homeostasis is a dynamic equilibrium.'

This property of living systems is very exciting to think about. Imagine a sailing ship on the oceans in the middle of a big storm with massive waves and high winds pushing and pulling it in all directions, and imagine that despite the rolling sideways and forwards and backwards she comes upright at every chance. Think about the body with emotional storms flooding through the systems while thoughts are directing actions of the limbs and digestive processes are taking place while breathing goes on.

Through all this the various physiological balances are maintained. Truly a magnificent achievement considering the enormous complexity and the billions of processes involved.

The intelligence must be awesome and the transfer of information must be happening at a most incredible rate. Again stop to consider who or what is in control.

Homeostasis suggests that there is both intelligence within the system and that the system has certain goalposts within which it functions. It is for this reason that weight reduction can be so difficult. The system may not have the same idea as the person regarding the weight it wants to balance at. Cut down calories and the metabolism slows down preventing any weight loss.

9: Self-Healing

It is so interesting that living systems should try and heal themselves. Non living systems tend to break down, to rust and have no way of renewal but living systems even in old age and despite the obvious degenerations and even when dying can still show signs of renewal and growth. Some livings systems can even regenerate tissue and even organs or grow limbs.

These are not small accomplishments because it again means that there is some intelligence at work, something that knows what 'normal' is and will move to return the system back to that 'normal' state.

The system must have a template or an image of self so that it constantly renews itself in a clearly defined way. Could aging be the fading or weakening of this image or template?

10: Systems Function Holistically

The word holistic is often misunderstood. It is not just about recognising that human beings are body plus mind plus spirit but rather that human beings are body/mind/spirit beings. There is no separation. Body is mind and mind is body. They are merely names for different functional aspects of the same living system.

Nothing in living systems functions on its own. Nothing can happen in one aspect of the system without the whole system responding. Disease may involve the part but in effect the whole system is affected and knows about it.

One cannot deal with the part in isolation. Treating with drugs which block the function of certain biochemical processes creates stress within the system. It is this stress which causes the side effects of drugs.

11: Living Systems are Intelligent

In many of the above examples I have referred to the presence of an intelligence which seems to be involved in the decision making and co-ordination of all processes within the system. In human beings this intelligence has a conscious and unconscious aspect, a voluntary and an involuntary aspect.   Even Darwin was impressed by this intelligence and wrote in the Origin of Species:

'....to suppose that the eye with all its inimitable contrivances for adjusting the focus to different distances, for admitting different amounts of light, and for the correction of spherical and chromatic aberration, could have been formed by natural selection, seems, I freely confess, absurd in the highest degree.'

Despite this his logical mind concluded that however sophisticated and despite the fact that he could not prove this, the development of the eye must have been due to natural selection.

The logical mind which can never see beyond its own logic concludes that what it does not understand does not exist. Science does the same thing and refuses to believe that which cannot be proved by scientific experiment and cannot be measured or weighed.

Intelligence is much more than logic however. Wisdom is not logical. Creativity does not always follow logical processes and can surprise the best scientists. There is inherent in living systems an intelligence which surprises, a response to stress and to challenge which is not mechanical but shows a uniqueness that is often awesome and will sometimes stretch the living system into new territory in its creativeness.

No scientist seems to be clear where this intelligence resides. The question of brain vs mind often comes up and whether animals and plants have minds or respond only in an instinctual way.

I believe there is intelligence within the human being and that this intelligence is vested in the mind, that the mind has its feet in the brain at one end and in a vaster consciousness at the other end. It is via consciousness that we all are connected . Consciousness also connect us to the animal and even plant world, to the past and future.

Consciousness<--->Mind<---> brain

There is a superb intelligence functioning within the system that at its very lowest level maintains body functions and at its highest levels sets goals and seeks beyond itself.

What does Systems Theory teach us?

- <u>That all things are connected</u>. The body-mind system is one whole and is not separate from the outer environment or the highest dimensions of spirit and soul.

- <u>There are no parts in a system.</u> In a compound there are no parts. The naming of functions, units and what appears as parts to the logical mind should not create the impression that these functions, units and apparent parts are independent of each other.

- <u>Mind and Body are not separate</u> but are names for two poles of the human being. There are other poles such as head and feet, right and left brain, inside and outside. None of the above are separate entities but represent only different ways in which we can describe the system that always remains whole and integrated.

- <u>Communication is Instantaneous.</u> This is absolutely necessary if the system is to survive. This suggests an informational transfer faster than the speed of light. This can only happen at the level of mind and not the physical world in which there is a limit to the speed with which information can travel.

- <u>Living Systems Maintain Balance and Harmony.</u> This balance and harmony appears to function within clearly defined limits called homeostasis.

Systems theory and the understanding of systems is essential to a more creative and fuller investigation of biological systems which are alive and functioning. Breaking systems up, separating and dividing, while useful is also limiting. It is essential that we understand the consequences of our actions so that we don't mistake the straw for the haystack or the sample of blood in the test tube for the person

Chapter 9

I have had a slight temperature for two days. Head feels a little foggy, nose blocked and then running mucus and a general malaise. Generally one likes to blame a virus for this cold and indeed a virus is always present but is it the cause or does it suggest a weak immune system is the primary problem? Naturopaths call a cold or flue a cleansing reaction i.e. my body is throwing out accumulated toxins that have reached critical levels and that this is a good thing. Spiritual seekers may regard the cold as having a much deeper meaning and not occurring in a haphazard way but bringing a message forward regarding the path ahead.

The argument over the cause of Aids suggests that establishing causes is not always straightforward. The dominant paradigm at the time will tend to overshadow all other explanations as to cause, nevertheless it behoves practitioners to listen carefully to what their patients believe is the cause and work with that as well.

The Causes of Ill Health

The conventional model of medicine tends to focus on the 'disease' and everything else becomes secondary and is often dismissed as unimportant.

'Our society and profession live by a view of science and reality that denies or belittles the reality of the subjective.

'Our life-stories are reduced to anecdotes. Our feelings are reduced to data that can be ignored. In the end our humanity is denied.'[1]

There is a whole range of other modalities and connections that are sidelined by the 'disease model' paradigm and these include the underlying dysfunction, which precedes the 'disease', the electromagnetic status of the biological system and any real focus on the underlying causes.

1   Fehrsen S Matter Mind and Medicine. Guest Editorial.
      Rod opi. 2000

In this chapter I want to focus on the underlying causes of disease. Many diseases are regarded as idiopathic (of unknown origin) and even when the causes are known, there is a tendency to dismiss the causes and just get on with the treatment of the disease.

The 'disease model' also leaves no time in the consultation for causes, which seems to be a confusing area. When the disease is so obvious, both doctor and patient are happy not to focus on the causes and taking responsibility for dealing with these causes becomes the responsibility of the patient if he or she wishes to go beyond just treating the disease with drugs.

Doctors may also lack understanding of causes, or themselves not follow a healthy lifestyle and therefore don't feel comfortable in discussing causes with their patients. For all these reasons lifestyle management and dealing with the causes of ill health tend to be sidetracked by most doctors.

Are the causes of ill health really unknown?

The causes of ill health are not really mysterious or unknown despite the fact that textbooks of medicine and conventional doctors will often claim that the cause of that particular disease has not yet been ascertained and is unknown or idiopathic.

Why do so many women have breast cancer and men have prostate cancer? What are the causes of heart disease, rheumatoid arthritis and the whole family of so called autoimmune diseases? The cause of these diseases and many others seem to be concealed behind a wall of confusion and a bewildering array of different points of view.

Allergic diseases are generally said to be caused by allergens, but if allergens are the cause of Hay fever and Asthma and other 'allergy' conditions, then how do we explain the fact that they do not cause problems in the majority of people exposed to them?

During an influenza epidemic only a certain proportion of the population becomes ill despite the fact that the whole population has never been exposed to this new virus. The ancient Greeks thought that disease was due to one of the four humours or elements, Fire, Air, Water and Earth.

In Traditional Chinese medicine the cause of disease is said to arise either from outside; usually one of the following weather conditions: cold, heat, damp, wind or summer i.e. from inside; usually emotional factors. Very often both emotional factors and external factors were involved.

In Ayurvedic medicine (traditional Indian medicine) lifestyle combined with a person's constitutional factors is important.

The history of modern medicine's battle with identifying the cause of ill health is of some interest. In 1856 Robert Koch, a very prominent microbiologist, claimed to have identified the cause of TB. Using a microscope and cell cultures he had identified what he claimed was a small microorganism. Not only did he identify this, the first microorganism, but also he laid the basis for the identification of microorganisms by other microbiologists. This became known as Koch's postulates.

There was much excitement in the medical community, as it seemed that at last the cause of many illnesses would be found to be other microorganisms. The race was on and over the next century thousands of microorganisms were discovered. Some of them could cause minor or even fatal diseases in human beings and animals.

About 80 years before Koch, Antoine Bechamp, regarded by many as the father of physiology, had suggested that the cause of ill health lay within the body itself. Ill health could only arise if the constitution was weak or the body had become weakened in some way. This susceptibility he claimed was the most important factor in the development of ill health.

Bechamp's theories however were soon supplanted by Koch's so that the medical profession turned to searching for causes outside the body and little attention was given to the innate resistance of the body to ill health. Instead the search for microorganisms in particular dominated medical research and is still regarded as an important avenue of research into the cause of ill health.

With the discovery of penicillin, pharmaceutical companies became established and the search for the magic bullet to cure all illness began. There are now scores of antibiotics and certainly they have saved untold number of lives, but does this prove that the bacteria they kill are the cause of ill health? Does the TB bacillus cause TB, the influenza virus cause influenza, the streptococcus cause tonsillitis and the staphylococcus cause boils? Are dust and pollens the cause of hay fever, milk the cause of some asthma and eczema?

A man has a serious argument with his wife and runs angrily out of the house. He is struck by lightning and dies. Autopsy reveals that he had a serious congenital condition of his heart.

It appears that the lightning is the immediate cause of the man's death, but would this have killed him if his heart was normal, if he was not angry? The argument with his wife had also resulted in him running out of the house. In this example we can see how complex it becomes when looking for single causes.

It should be clear from the above review that the cause of illness is not simply due to a single factor. Microorganism are only one component of the problem, there must be susceptibility also. The human beings that contract a cold or flue are the ones that are vulnerable. If it was merely the presence of bacteria or viruses then hospitals would be exceedingly dangerous places and doctors and nurses would be dying at a rapid rate.

No single cause of ill health.

The causes are complex and effects depend on the body's susceptibility. We now have two components regarding the cause of ill health. There are factors from outside i.e. microorganism or allergens and factors from inside the system, which create susceptibility so that the outside factors can precipitate ill health. Two examples will clarify the issues involved and allow us to move on.

The Mercedes Benz does not come out of the factory 100% perfect, but does not break down immediately. In time however various weaknesses begin to emerge. These weaknesses are exposed and aggravated by the conditions of the road travelled daily, the tyre pressure, the quality of the petrol and oil used, the driving technique and the general way the driver looks after the car.

One day it goes over a bump in the road and something breaks. What are we going to blame, the bump, the driver, the weather, petrol, oil or the factory? Obviously all these factors had a part to play and no one factor can be blamed. The bump in the road was the precipitating factor.

Similarly with ill health in human beings, the virus, bacteria or allergen can be regarded as the precipitating factor rather than the cause, just as the bump in the road was the straw that broke the camel's back. Without the background of change, which had weakened the system, the motorcar would not have broken down. Similarly without the susceptibility in the body, the micro-organism would not have been able to cause any infection. Both the precipitating factors and the susceptibility are important in the development of ill health.

It is of special interest that when a child, for example, develops an infection, it usually involves one micro-organism despite the fact that there are hundreds of possible organism that can precipitate ill health. Is there a possible lock and key effect here in which only one organism can fit into the susceptible space? The key that fits into a lock has a very special shape and only a key with that shape fits into that lock. I suspect that there may be a similar condition at work here i.e. the 'shape' of the susceptibility and the 'shape' of the micro-organism must fit.

Persons who have recurrent bladder infections or recurrent middle ear infections or recurrent infections of any kind, have a specific susceptibility and in general the same microorganism tends to be involved. Something similar happens with allergies. The susceptibility is usually to very specific substances or allergens.

Lock and key effect between the outside factors and internal susceptibility.

I will be discussing the how and the why of the susceptible space in other chapters, but for the moment the underlying causes of illness is our focus of attention. We have identified two main groups of causes:

- The precipitating cause or causes
- The susceptible space in the system

In general the susceptible space must first develop and this may be enough for ill health to manifest. In other words, no precipitating factor is necessary; the weakness in the system is enough to cause symptoms and signs of ill health to slowly develop. An example would be the patient complaining of tiredness or even heart disease. There may be no obvious precipitating factors, but the patient continues to become more and more ill.

What is the cause of this susceptibility to ill health?

In the example of the motorcar there were three basic factors involved and these have equivalence in the human system:

- The motor car did not come out of the factory perfect.

Human beings do not emerge from the factory perfect either.

= Genetic factors

The motor is subject to environmental factors;

- Petrol, oil, road conditions, weather etc.

- The human being is subject to food, water, air, electromagnetic fields, geopathic stress, microorganisms, pollution, etc.

= Environmental factors,

There are good drivers and bad drivers

= Emotional/mental factors

Persons with ill health, who have journeyed through the portals of conventional medicine going from one doctor to another seeking a cause and cure for their illness, may become even more confused travelling the corridors of those practitioners involved in natural medicine.

- The chiropractor may blame their problem on a misalignment of their spine.

- The reflexologist may discover tender points over the liver, adrenals and lung points in the soles of the feet and blame the problem on a dysfunction of these organs.

- The naturopath may suggest that the patient's ill health was caused by an acid condition of the blood requiring a change of diet.

- Other practitioners may blame Candida.

- The new age psychotherapist may suggest that the deep seated root of the ill health is a spiritual one and required various psychotherapeutic techniques; including hypnosis and visualization exercises.

As the person journeys from one practitioner to the other they may begin to wonder if anyone really knows what is going on or eventually they find someone whose explanation makes sense to them and this will be confirmed if they begin to feel better as a result of the treatment. I have seen patients stay with a doctor whose explanation makes sense even for years despite the fact that the condition has not improved.

Multiple causes – multiple explanations

But what is the truth?

The Causes of Ill Health

Is conventional medicine all wrong, because their medication generally treats symptoms only, requiring patients to take these drugs for years or even indefinitely? Is the natural way always preferable and closer to the truth in terms of understanding causes? Yet there seems to be a constant proliferation of new ideas and different emphasis on causes.

There was a time when my investigation into different methods of treatment and different philosophies brought me to a point of exasperation and frustration. It seemed that all philosophies had their adherents and practitioners specialising in the various methods. All had their successes and failures despite the difference in philosophies and methods of treatment.

Slowly, with time and as my own successes and failures gave me more understanding, there was the realization that there is a basic underlying truth that helped me make sense of what was happening. It is this truth, a basic principle, which is at work that I would like to share with all those reading this book. Let me first state these principles and then explain them:

- There is no single cause for any ill health

- The causes leave imprints/dysfunction within the biological system

- These imprints/dysfunction may be of minor or major significance

- A minor imprint/ dysfunction may however precipitate a major illness, 'The straw that breaks the camel's back.'

- The biological system has the ability to 'contain', 'store' or 'control' for months or years these imprints without producing major distortion of function.

- Eventually the pressure of these imprints/dysfunctions reaches a critical mass and the pressure build up runs along the lines of least resistance within the system causing a crack to appear.

- The crack is a release valve and is usually considered 'the disease'. I sometimes refer to the crack as the 'end point'.

- The cause of the 'crack/end point' is the underlying combination of imprints/dysfunction.

What exactly are these imprints/dysfunction and where are they stored and why do I refer to them as both an 'imprint' on the one hand and a 'dysfunction' on the other?

When one presses one's hand onto a pane of glass an imprint remains behind when the hand is removed. In a similar way informational imprints, which interfere with function, appear in the biological system. This may be similar to viruses in a computer.

As indicated in previous chapter on the anatomy of man / woman, human beings are not just physical structures with biochemical processes but have various energetic bodies. It is here that these imprints are stored and are not detected by the tools of conventional medicine. Thus a person may have severe symptoms with extreme tiredness, headaches and loss of appetite and weight yet all tests may be normal.

Some of the newer electromagnetic tools used by certain health practitioners claim to detect these imprints. When the electromagnetic disturbance affects biochemical functions then 'dysfunction' in biochemistry begins to appear. Please review the chapter on the 'human anatomy revisited'.

Case study

Mrs M.S. has had recurrent severe headaches for years. She is seldom without headaches and treats herself with 2-6 pain pills per day. At least once per month she needs an anti- inflammatory injection from her local general practitioner. She has been to a number of specialists, but all investigations including an MRI scan have been normal. Physiotherapy, chiropractic adjustment and even reflexology have been helpful for a short time only. A course of acupuncture treatment eventually gave her substantial relief and she was able to stop analgesia treatment.

Comment: Despite the severity of the headache, all tests were normal. How do we explain this phenomenon?

A person has a motorcar, which is not functioning well. She has had the motorcar for many years and is familiar with its 'feel', sound of the engine and the way it rides and is certain that it needs to be fixed. The mechanic looks through the motorcar carefully and finds nothing wrong.

'Madam,' he says, 'I have given your motor a very good examination and I believe there is nothing mechanically wrong with it.'

The woman, who is convinced that there is problem, asks the mechanic to please drive the car around the block, which he agrees to do rather reluctantly. When he returns however, he has to agree with the lady that in fact there is definitely something wrong.

What has happened is something very simple and which I see almost daily. Ill feeling patients go to doctors insisting that there must be something wrong only to be told by their doctor that nothing is wrong, it must be all in their imagination, or stress only.

When the motor is standing still in the garage with the engine off, nothing wrong can be found. When, however the mechanic drives the car, he can hear and feel what the owner of the car noted. The car is obviously not broken; otherwise the mechanic would have found this on examination. When it is only out of tune however, this cannot be 'diagnosed' unless the car was being driven around.

Similarly it is most unfair for doctors to tell patients who are complaining of symptoms that nothing is wrong just because all the tests are normal. If the system is out of tune only, then all tests may also be normal. To say that the biological system is 'out of tune' suggests its function is abnormal.

A person with chronic headaches has a system out of tune unless there is something physically detectable such as a brain tumour. This is then an 'end point' diagnosis. The system has moved from 'out of tune' to 'breakdown'.

It is possible therefore that the disturbance is primarily at the level of the energy fields of the patient and only secondary some disturbance in physiology. This explains why acupuncture, a relaxation technique or a simple compassionate hand on the shoulder may alleviate the problem.

Conventional medical doctors use testing i.e. X-rays, biochemistry and biopsy to make a diagnosis of disease while Integrative Health practitioners tend to use testing in order to make a diagnosis of functional disturbances and to identify underlying causes.

The mechanic knew the car was out of tune mainly from the "feel" and sound of the engine, much like a piano tuner tunes the piano. The patient complains that something is wrong and yet the doctor assures her that nothing is wrong, because all tests are normal. It is not uncommon for the system to be "out of tune" for prolonged periods, even months or years and then only have a 'breakdown' with a severe stress factor or stress which may reach a critical mass leading to the breakdown

Functional Disturbance/Disease out of Tune - - -> Breakdown/ the disease

The system has an enormous reservoir of adaptabilities so that despite the functional disturbance, it can maintain normal function for a very long time with only minor symptoms and signs until eventually breakdown occurs and the 'disease' manifests.

Summary

There is no single cause to ill health. Plants, animals, human beings are all subject to multiple factors which could lead to ill health.

Each person has a unique background of biological factors maintaining health and preventing ill health. This is the physical body's resistance and includes the immune function, genetic factors, constitutional factors, hormonal factors and the general function of all the organs and systems and the way they work together. Other factors less well understood include inner peace, mindfulness and spiritual fortitude which all may influence the resistance to ill health.

Multiple factors work against health both from the external environment and internal causes. In the background is the 'energy-informational' aspects of the human greater anatomy where imprints and energy disturbances occur and may work there way into physiology and eventually anatomy. The relationship between the internal resistance and the factors working against this defines whether the person becomes ill or not.

The Causes

In my experience most patients are pretty clear why they have become ill and don't usually need much prompting. Their reasons may sometimes seem obscure to the doctor, either because of the cultural differences or because of the subjective nature of the causes.

Nevertheless doctors need to be aware of how thinking and emotions stir up physiological effects. Both the placebo and nocebo responses are extremely powerful ways that mind can influence the body in the short and long term.

There are a number of diseases that have 'lifestyle problem' written all over them, and the two common ones are cardiovascular disease and diabetes type 2 (DM2). Both these diseases have increased dramatically over the last decade to become among the most common causes of morbidity and mortality.

Myocardial infarction was almost unknown before the turn of this century, and has become the number one killer. A number of studies with angiographic confirmation have shown reversal of narrowing in the coronary arteries with lifestyle changes. In 1999 the peer reviewed journal 'Circulation' carried an article reporting that people who had already had one heart attack and followed a Mediterranean diet had a 70% reduction in all-cause mortality compared to controls.[234]

Most causes will fit under one of the following headings:

- Genetic
- Poor food choices
- Lack of exercise
- Obesity
- Toxins in the environment
- Micro-organisms, fungi, parasites.
- Injury
- Stress
- Poor sleep patterns
- Electromagnetic pollution

2   Lorgeril de Michel et al Mediterranean Diet, Traditional risk factors & the rate of cardiovascular complications after myocardial infarction. Circulation. 1999
3 Ornish D et al Can lifestyle changes reverse coronary heart disease? The Lifestyle heart trial.Lancet 336 (8708): 129-33

4   Blankenhorn Can atherosclerotic lesions regress? Angiographic evidence in humans. Am J Cardio 1990;65(12):41F-43F

- Drugs
- Xeno-estrogens
- Nutritional deficiencies

Genetics

No motorcar comes out of the factory 100% perfect; nevertheless the car does not break down immediately but over time as it is subject to environmental conditions. The same applies to every human being born today.

Subtle differences in genetic factors cause people to respond differently when exposed to the same environmental factors. It is becoming clear today that environmental factors can make all the difference in how the genes respond and this accounts for the fact that individuals in the same family with a genetic disturbance don't develop exactly the same presentation of that disease, nor at the same age.

All diseases probably have a genetic component, which cannot necessarily be changed, but the expression and the way those genes function are dependent on the food consumed and even exercise and stress can make a difference to that expression.

The science of 'nutrigenomics' is the study of how foods affect our genes and how individual genetic differences can affect the way we respond to nutrients (and other naturally occurring compounds) in the food we eat.

Certain foods and nutrients such as vitamin D for example can both promote good expression of the genetic potential if adequate amounts present or prevent or distort normal genetic expression if insufficient.

Optimum genetic function also requires a range of nutrients to maintain health and other nutrients (antioxidants) to protect the DNA from damage due to free radicals and toxins.

Genetics may limit what functions can happen in the body but the full expression of body functions is dependent on environmental factors.

Food Choices

There is probably no single diet suitable for everyone. Food choices should take into account that the foods we eat certainly contain the building blocks for bodybuilding and repair, but food also contains immune stimulating properties, antioxidant properties, antimicrobial properties, anti-inflammatory properties, anticancer properties and detoxification properties. Food also steers the body towards a more alkaline or acid environment.

Diet should be based on whole foods (vegetables, fruits and fibre), preferably organic and fresh. Onions, garlic and cold-pressed olive oil are all healthy. Meat should be from free-range grass-fed animals and fish should be from a natural sea environment rather than farmed fish, eaten a few times per week. Processed and junk food should be excluded. This would include processed oils (most oils not cold pressed), margarine and any food containing trans fats.

Mediterranean vs. low fat diet:

The Mediterranean diet can lower the risk of heart disease, stroke and chances of dying from many diseases by 30%. In a study[5] of 7500 men and women ages 55-80 years, none had heart disease at the beginning of study but all had heart disease risk factors. Some smoked, half had diabetes, and most were overweight with high BP and high cholesterol levels.

No calorie restriction and no exercise were required. They ate either a low-fat diet or Mediterranean diet which included three daily servings of fruit and veg along with fish and legumes at least 3x/week with an either an extra tablespoon daily of mixed nuts or a generous handful of almonds, walnuts and/or hazelnuts, or four extra tablespoons of extra-virgin olive oil. A glass of wine with meals was allowed but not required. No junk food or sweets were allowed, and red and processed meats were discouraged.

The study was stopped early because of the results: a 30% drop in heart attacks and strokes in those on the Mediterranean diet. Few people stayed on the low-fat diet, so the study ended up comparing the Mediterranean diet to a typical western diet.

5   Estruch R et al PREDIMED study investi- gators.
     Primary prevention of cardiovascular disease with
     Med diet NEJM 2013; 368: 1279- 1290

What about the high fat diet (Banting, Ketogenic) so popular today?

I am generally not in favour of food choices that require too much effort and a constant attention to detail. These high fat diets make absolute sense to me and have a very particular place in my practice of medicine and supporting healing.

The body can use two sources of food for energy that is either glucose from carbohydrates or ketones produced from fat. If lots of carbohydrates are not available then the body uses fat in foods to produce ketones but it can also use the fat stored in the body.

Reducing carbs in the diet would result in the body drawing ketones from the fat stored. This then is an easy way for most people to lose weight rapidly. In my experience most people, but not all, will lose a great deal of weight if they go on a high fat, low carb and medium protein diet. This is not a high protein diet, which is probably not healthy and very acidic.

The medical profession has resisted shifting their stance on their recommended standard western diet with its heavy emphasis on at least 50% carbohydrates, even if it does include whole grains rather than refined grains, and continue to deny the value of fat in the diet. The Standard American Diet which includes cheeseburgers, French fries, super-sized sodas, pizzas, doughnuts, pancakes and often lots of charcoaled meats has generated the epidemic of obesity and diabetes and may have a high fat content but most of the fats are processed and include trans fats with their carcinogenic potential.

I do not suggest people follow the high fat diet long term unless they have epilepsy or certain cancers such as brain cancer, which definitely responds to this diet. My feeling is that we need more long-term studies and that this diet may not be appropriate for everyone.

My preference is for the Mediterranean style diet with lots of organic vegetables and fruit, free range meats, sea water fish, cold pressed oils, nuts and seeds and whole grains in those able to tolerate grains. Raw milk and products made from raw milk may work for some people as well. Buffalo or goats milk and products may be a better choice than cow's milk because the animals have had fewer drugs fed to them.

Choose a diet that does not make you obsessive about what you eat.

Choose healthy farm fresh foods.

Lack of Exercise

Our ancestors and contemporary hunter-gatherers walked an average of 10 000 steps (about 10 km) per day, with frequent bouts of more intense physical activity. Even in more recent times people where not couch potatoes sitting all day in front of TV and computers but were more involved in manual labour. All this has changed over the last 50 years. Even children do much less activity and play less outdoors, spending more time sitting.

People now spend an average of six hours a day sitting and often even more time in the evening. We were not genetically designed to sit all day and science is showing that sitting too much shortens our lifespans.

In an Australian study that followed participants over six-and-a-half years, researchers found that high levels of TV time were significantly associated with increased risk of death from heart disease as well as all other causes. Each hour increment of TV viewing was associated with an 11 percent increase in death from all causes[6].

By contrast, those who watched less than two hours of TV a day had a 46 percent lower risk of death from all causes when compared to those who watched more than four hours. These associations were independent of exercise and traditional risk factors such as smoking, blood pressure, cholesterol levels, waist circumference, and diet. It seems that sitting too long is as risky as smoking and that all the exercise one may do may not compensate for too much sitting.

Toxins

The environment today abounds with toxins of all kinds. Many of the toxins used in industry and even in food production have not been fully evaluated for human consumption, but invariably filter into the human body. Heavy metals such as lead, mercury and cadmium have no known beneficial role in human metabolism, and are extremely toxic in high and even low doses.

6   Dunstand DW et al Television viewing time and mortality. Circulation.2010;121(3)

They are ubiquitous in industrialised countries but also find their way to the furthest corners of the planet via wind and water. While some countries have specified lower limits of normal in the blood, the fact is that many doctors believe that there are no normal limits, and that even very low levels over time can cause serious disease.

One needs to take into account the fact that heavy metals are present in the body in various combinations with other toxins, a background of genetic polymorphism, food combinations that support or interfere with elimination, fatty liver, leaky gut, immune system compromised etc., which can aggravate the problem in certain individuals, and this is why one person can tolerate much higher levels of toxins than another.

In one study[7], for example, blood lead levels of 13 956 adults who were part of the Third National Health and Nutrition Examination Survey were examined. They were recruited from 1988 to 1994 and followed up for 12 years.

The goal was to track which diseases people developed and why they died. Fifty years ago the average blood level was 40mcg/dl; now less than 10mcg/dl is considered normal.

In this study researchers found that a level of lead over 2mcg/dl caused dramatic increases in heart attacks, strokes and death. After controlling for other risk factors, including cholesterol, high BP, smoking and inflammation, there was still a risk from all causes in people with high levels of lead.

Death from heart disease increased by 55%, risk of heart attacks increased by 151% and risk of stroke increased by 89%. Nearly 40% of American's are estimated to have blood levels of lead high enough to cause these problems

High blood pressure in postmenopausal women is strongly correlated to blood lead levels.

Lead is connected to the epidemic of children with ADHD, developmental and learning problems and autism. Studies show a drop off in IQ scores in children occurs in those who have lead levels between 1 and 10mcg/dl.

7   Menke A et al Blood lead below 10mcg/dl and mortality among US adults. 2006 Circulation 114(13): 1388-94

Mercury has similar problems[8]. The relatively high solubility of certain mercury salts in water enables them to be readily taken up and bio-transformed to methyl mercury by certain fish. This is a major source of mercury exposure in humans.

Mercury exerts it toxic effects by competing with and displacing iron and copper from the active sites of enzymes involved in energy production. This induces mitochondrial dysfunction and oxidative damage.

Cadmium, on the other hand, mimics zinc and disrupts zinc metabolism. Zinc is essential for immune function. Other metals, which can be toxic, include iron, aluminum and copper.

Metals are only one group of toxins in the environment. Other chemicals also disrupt biochemical pathways, block or even activate receptor sites (e.g. xeno-estrogens) and act as competitive antagonists to vitamins, minerals and co-factors of enzyme function.

Measuring the level of toxins may still miss the effect of synergy, that is when toxins are combined in low doses there may still be a synergistic toxic effect of the whole.

Drugs are a major cause of ill health and even death, now recognised to be the 3rd or 4th most common cause of ill health and death, with some researchers suggesting that if all the negative effects were reported, iatrogenic (doctor induced) disease would be the most common cause of morbidity and mortality.

Check out chapter 10 on the toxic environment.

Obesity

Obesity is the leading cause of preventable deaths in the USA and is often associated with diabetes, leading to the diagnosis of Diabesity. Diabesity will affect 1 in 2 Americans by the year 2020 and 90% of these will not be diagnosed. Gaining 5 to 7,2kg doubles the risk of DM2. In South Africa it is estimated that 1 in 5 children is either overweight or obese.

8   Houston MC Role of mercury toxicity in hypertension, cardiovascular disease, and stroke..J Clin Hypertens(Greenwich) 2011; 13(8):621-7

One in three children born today will have diabetes in their lifetime. Rates are increasing worldwide:

In China the rate of diabetes was almost zero 25 years ago; by 2007 there were 24 million diabetics and by 2010 there were 93 million diabetics and 148 million pre-diabetics.

In the Middle East nearly 20-25% of the population is diabetic.

Doctors are starting to see young children with type 2 diabetes and adult complications of Metabolic Syndrome in children.

Our Paleolithic ancestors ate the equivalent of 22 teaspoons of sugar per year.

At the beginning of the 1800s, the average person consumed 4.5kg a year. Today, the average American eats 68 to 82kg per year.

A 600ml sweetened carbonated drink or sports drink contains 17 teaspoons of sugar.

With all this information it is not rocket science deciding what the underlying cause of metabolic syndrome, obesity and DM2 and cardiovascular disease is. But what needs to shift is the 'disease paradigm' where the emphasis is on treating the 'end point' (the disease) rather than really focusing on the underlying causes. These include lack of exercise, refined foods and excess sugar consumption.

Heart disease can also be reversed by much more focus on lifestyle by the medical profession and health departments, which tend to be overwhelmed by the need to treat the diseases of AIDS, TB and diabetic complications.

Health clinics, which are really 'disease clinics', should have 'health clinics' attached, where people can be taught lifestyle management skills. Health departments need to turn their attention, towards promoting healthy eating habits, in the same way they have with cigarette smoking, and place increasing limits on junk food.

Stress

Many studies have shown that stress increases the incidence of ill health and that stress management has a significant role in improving health.

Living alone after a heart attack for example more than doubles the risk of dying in the first year after a heart attack.[9]

Stress management components include meditation, breathing exercises; walking one's pet daily, supportive family and friends, various relaxation techniques, psychotherapy etc.

Pollution

3.5 to 4.5 kg of chemicals, which the physical body has never had to deal with before, are consumed by the average American every year. This is a massive invasion and a real burden to the body's defense and detox systems. A large percentage of these chemicals are known carcinogens and are associated with depression, memory decline, asthma, eczema, migraine, irritable bowel and many other serious diseases including Parkinson's disease, Multiple Sclerosis and in fact any chronic disease will have some toxic chemical as one of the underlying causes.

The background of toxins and the synergistic aspects of the combination of multiple toxins and their effects on the body are almost impossible to calculate. Toxins interfere with function and poor function only aggravates and compound the harm that is being done.

Many of these toxins have estrogenic like effects by fitting into the estrogen receptor. These are called xeno-estrogens and may be contributing to the increased incidence of breast cancer, prostate cancer and infertility.

Toxins are present in the food we eat especially in processed foods, in the water we drink and in the air we breathe. It is not possible to escape completely the toxic load but every effort should be made to reduce the load by using filtered water, organic non-processed foods and by living away from seriously polluted air. If you can smell chemicals then they are entering your body. Really not a good idea to work in such an environment.

9   Gullette et al. Effects of mental stress on myocardial ischemia during daily life. JAMA 1997 277:1521-1526.

Poor sleep patterns

Millions of people suffer from insomnia while others just work their life away and are too busy to even go to sleep. Research has shown that too little sleep and even too much sleep is not good for one's health.

In the USA it was estimated that 100,000 crashes on the road are due to drivers falling asleep at the wheel. Even children can have problems falling asleep and this is often due to spending too much time sitting in front of bright lights (computers, TV screens or any other source of bright light) in the hour before going to bed.

There are natural biorhythms that are governed by hormone shifts and the melatonin increase at night to induce sleep requires darkness. This is a biological imperative and can be disturbed by the night becoming as bright as the day. It is a good idea therefore to turn down the light and read children bedtime stories rather than let them watch highly charged TV or other programmes before bed.

Chronic insomniacs are more likely that others to develop psychiatric problems, such as depression or anxiety disorder, skill solving becomes slowed down and risk taking tends to increase.

Long-term sleep deprivation may increase the severity of chronic disease including high blood pressure and diabetes. Studies have also shown that the longer it takes to fall asleep and more times the individual wakes up during the night, the more severe the hypertension.

Caffeine is clearly a stimulant and can keep people awake but what is less well known is that it takes 15-35 hours for the caffeine to leave the body after consumption. This is my personal experience. Taking coffee anytime from 12 midday can cause me to have a coffee insomnia that night. Insomniacs are also more sensitive to the effects of coffee.

Not getting enough sleep may also lead to weight gain and big boost in calorie intake thus promoting obesity.

'Sleep is essential and healthy sleep should be as important as healthy nutrition, physical activity and smoking cessation in promoting overall health.'[10]

Conclusion

The information above is only an introduction to the causative field of ill health. It emphasises the role of poor food choices, lack of exercise and sleep, being overweight, toxins in the environment and stress. Many other factors are mentioned whose role may still be controversial, such as electromagnetic exposure.

The work of Robert Becker[11] and Robert Liburdy[12] still reverberates through the research community. The commercial, legal and financial consequences of any documented link between electromagnetic exposure and cancer however is enormous, and these works tend to be ignored and kept out of the public arena.

The psychological components of ill health should not be dismissed either. The placebo and nocebo effects are powerful indicators of the power of our intention, attitudes and the emotional components of our lives. Most patients know this and don't appreciate it when doctors cast doubt or dismiss these factors when a diagnosis of cancer or Parkinson's disease, for example, is made. People can be chronically stressed, and this places enormous pressure on every system of the body.

The ability of the doctor to change the patient's story from one that does not work for them ('poor me', 'I'm not good enough', 'I'll never get better') to a story that supports the way they want to feel about themselves will leave a deep impression on that patient. The story the

10 Wheaton A, et al 'Sleep disordered breathing and depression among U.S. adults: National Health and Nutrition Examination Survey, 2005-2008' Sleep 2012; 35: 1-7.

11 Becker RO Cross Currents: The promise of Electromedicine. The perils of electropollution. Penguin group, Inc New York 1990

12   Liburdy RP Wyant A Radiofrequency radi- ation and the immune system. Int J Radiat Biol Stud Phys Chem Med 1984; 46(1): 67-81

patient has about himself or herself can promote ill health or turn ill health around.

Doctors have an important role in gaining insight into possible causes of disease. This is not usually that difficult. Lifestyle can be assessed from questionnaires given to the patient before they enter the consulting room, and with a few key questions patients will open up to the doctor.

Clearly a five-minute consultation is not nearly adequate, but then doctors need to decide whether they are interested in the health of their patients, or just a symptomatic approach using drugs. Healthy changes to lifestyle will start a healing process.

A medicine where the emphasis is on healing the person is superior to a medicine where doctors take out the prescription pad the moment the patient walks into the consulting room in order to treat the disease.

Chapter 10

Standing in the aisle of the supermarket waiting my turn to pay is always quite an eye opener for me as I see what people are buying for their family. The poorer the person the less full the basket and more refined cheap quality foods are being bought. The richer the person the more full the basket but nevertheless most of the food and other items are still processed, frozen, synthetic and junk foods to appese the taste buds but not to nourish the body. Wine, coke, sweets, white bread, buns, cakes, chemically derived cleaning solutions, poison sprays, fruit juice and lots of meat and chicken which are not free range. How our diet has changed over 100 years and even from when I was a child.

The Toxic Environment

Cancer is now a killing and disabling disease of epidemic proportions. In 2012 there were 14.1 million new cases world wide with 8.2 million cancer deaths and 32.6 million people living with cancer.

Cancer poses a major threat to public health worldwide, and incidence rates have increased in most countries since 1990. The trend is a particular threat to developing nations with health systems that are ill-equipped to deal with complex and expensive cancer treatments putting enormous strain on government and public health agencies, insurance companies, public taxes, hospitals and clinics.

The war against cancer is very far from being won, with no obvious solution in sight. Yet despite constant denial from the medical establishment, there is good evidence that the cause of cancer is not the mystery that most people assume and are led to believe.

In 1900 the leading causes of death were influenza, pneumonia, and gastroenteritis, followed by heart disease and cerebral haemorrhage. Cancer was number 8 and caused less than 4% of all deaths. By 1976 cancer was the second leading cause of death after heart disease, accounting for 20% of all deaths, a percentage that is still increasing.

It is expected that cancer will soon become the leading cause of death with every second person dying from cancer. With the increase so obviously related to the last 100 years there is a need to consider a possible cause within the environment.

Cancer is not the only illness that has increased at a rapid rate and continues to increase in incidence with each decade. Allergy problems have almost doubled in the last 15 years from 10 to 20% of children now suffer from some form of allergy. Type 2 diabetes has increased at an astonishing rate as has auto-immune disease.

'We have no other good explenation as to why there should be an increase in autoimmune diseases, except for the things to which we are exposed in the environment. Autoimmunity is our immune system's effort to adapt to all the new environmental agents and shifts that we're being bombarded with. It's an unsuccessful adaptation, but it's our body's way of trying to fight back.'[1]

Although many doctors may blame hereditary factors for these increases, common sense would suggest that this is highly unlikely. Genetic changes just do not occur over such short periods of time unless these doctors are referring to direct damage to genetic material by poisons or radiation.

What has happened very clearly over the last 100years is changing eating patterns on the one hand and especially the enormous increase in pollution and poisons in the environment, many which are now recognised as carcinogens.

Statistics show that tobacco kills more people than AIDS, drugs, accidents and alcohol together. In the USA alone, there are 430 000 tobacco related deaths annually which results in more than $50 billion in direct medical costs. There appears to be hundreds of chemical compounds in cigarette smoke many which are now recognised to be carcinogens while the total load of chemicals can also suppress the immune system and damage the lung tissue.

In a study reported in the British Medical Journal (2000,320:53) it was shown that a smokers life span was reduced by 6.5 years or as much as 11 minutes for every cigarette smoked. The high incidence of cancer of the mouth in Asia, representing some 35% of all Asiatic cancers, is clearly due to the common habit of chewing betel nuts and tobacco leaves.

Chemicals can clearly cause ill health and so can radiation and yet researchers continue to search for the cause of cancer as if it is not

1 Noel R. Rose MD, PhD Director, Autoimmune Disease Research Center, John Hpkins Medical Institution.

obviously on their doorstep. This is not to suggest that all cancers are due to toxins or radiation because as has already been dealt with in other chapters all ill health has multiple causes but certainly these toxins are a major contributory factor and may even be the deciding factor in the particular mode of expression of that particular combination of causes.

Environmental Chemicals cause Ill Health and Death

Of great concern to the average person is the increase in the number of new chemicals over which we have no control. Smoking can be stopped and so can betel chewing, but there is a whole range of new chemicals filtering into the food chain and environment over which there seems to be little control. Of particular concern are the following factors:

- Chemicals introduced in foods but not appearing on labels. Very often these chemicals are still regarded as inert or non-poisonous or in too small a dose to have any untoward effects.

- Chemicals in the environment which are allowed because the benefits outweigh the risks. An example of this is chlorine and fluoride introduced into the drinking water. Both chlorine and fluoride are byproducts of industry and highly poisonous. Chlorine is used to disinfect water i.e. to kill micro-organism while fluoride was introduced to decrease the caries in teeth of children.

If chlorine disinfects water then one must understand that it will do the same in the gastro-intestinal tract i.e. kill or inhibit some of the body's own micro-organism. It is not at all clear what the long-term consequences of this would be. It seems that there is little money for this kind of research.

No government wants to start worrying about changing the way water is sanitised when a system seems to be working, so from the government's point of view the risks are worth the benefits. Chlorine is converted into chloride in the body and while this is not toxic it is what happens to chlorine in the presence of organic material that is particularly dangerous and toxic.

Chlorine forms Disinfection Byproducts (DBPs) which are a hundred times more toxic than chlorine. While the level of chlorine present in drinking water is regarded as safe, the fact is that chlorine water and its byproducts are present in numerous other sources such as drinks and foods grown in chlorinated water.

Americans ingest from 300 to 600 times what the Environmental Protection Agency considers a 'safe' amount. Chlorine and its byproducts are carcinogenic and add to the total load of carcinogens in the environment. Don't expect any government to change this. You will be told that the benefits far outweigh the risks.

Fluoride poured into drinking water may even turn out to be a bigger scam than chlorine. There is insufficient data regarding the safe daily intake over the long term. Although the possibility of toxic effects is dismissed by government agencies and most medical scientists as insignificant, one cannot dismiss the fact that fluoride is a poison and that with time the total amount of fluoride in the environment will increase.

This increase will follow the increasing amounts appearing in watered plants and trees and eventually in fruit, vegetables and even animal tissue. This increase will eventually filter down into the tissues of human beings who eat and drink contaminated foods and water. While there may be a level of control around the amount of fluoride present in the water, the accumulated traces of fluoride eventually ending up in the food eaten is very difficult to control.

Chlorine and Fluoride are Chemical Poisons

The effect of synergy.

Synergism: The action of two or more substances to achieve an effect of which each is individually incapable.

Synergy is extremely important yet almost no research scientist even attempts to enter this arena of research because of the enormous complexity. Why is synergy important?

• When two or more substances/chemicals are mixed together there is often an enhanced effect. It is as if each substance contributes to enhancing the effects of the other. Selenium and Vitamin E for example appear to have a synergistic effect, which is useful, but chemicals that may not appear to have harmful effects in the dose range used may become poisonous when combined with other chemicals.

• Arising from the above one must therefore conclude that when mixing chemicals much lower doses may be necessary to produce the same effects and prevent poisoning. Despite this understanding doctors often prescribe multiple drugs without being clear what the synergistic effect will be in that patient and governments and other agencies mix chemicals in a haphazard way in foods, water and drinks without any research regarding the consequences of this mixing on human beings and other living systems.

• The scenario is complicated even more when we consider how the chemical mix from outside meets the biochemical soup within the human body. The synergy and suppression of function is impossible to predict.

No chemical is an island entire to itself but becomes part of each living system into which it enters. Tobacco is a risk factor for cancer of the lung. Adding asbestos multiplies the risk many fold, much more than one would expect from each individually. Pesticides have been shown to amplify one another's toxicity by 500-1000 fold.[2]

What does this mean to all of us exposed to such large amounts of different pesticides and other chemicals? In 1945, the USA annual production of chemicals was 8 million tons and this rose to 110 million tons by 1985. This is approximately 950lbs of chemicals for each person in the USA.

• Chemical mimics in the environment and food chain. These are referred to as 'Xenotoxins' and can function as the body's own intrinsic chemical substances. A good example is the group of substances known as Xenohormones. These are substances found in nature, which have hormonal effects. Many of these hormone-like substances are found in solvents, adhesives, petrochemical products, car exhaust, plastics, industrial waste, meat from livestock fed estrogenic drugs to fatten them up and synthetic hormones. Think of little girls playing with finger nail polish, men and woman working in dry cleaning places, exposed to paint and varnish, cleaning products and hobby material. The Xenohormones are poisonous and interfere with the delicate hormonal balance by blocking receptor sites because of their similarity to the natural hormones. There is also the additive and synergistic effect together with the cumulative long-term effects with many of these chemicals, which are not biodegradable and build up in the fatty tissues of the body.

With this enormous increase of xenohormones in the environment has come the increasing incidence of breast cancer and prostate cancer.

2   Arnold SF et al. Science.vol 272. p1489. 1996

There is sufficient evidence that estrogens are carcinogenic arising from their cell stimulating effects and chronic exposure may also be responsible for the rise in infertility problems.

Infertility and cancer have been increasing exponentially with the increasing pollution of the environment. Looking for genetic causes and micro-organism as causes for cancer seems to be a way of deviating time and money away from the major factors in this serious illness. One wonders how serious researchers are in wanting to find the real cause.

I am listing below some of the pollutant in our environment, which could be contributing to the increasing incidence of ill health. This is only a small sample to give one an insight into the vast arena of this polluted world.

Amalgam Fillings

Amalgam fillings, which contain mainly mercury and silver and used to fill cavities in teeth. Although dentists and government bodies refuse to acknowledge the possibility that these substances in amalgams could be dangerous to one's health there is sufficient data to suggest that traces of mercury are in fact leaking from these fillings due to the constant action of chewing and the digestive action of saliva.

Many different metals are often used to fill cavities and there is a measurable electrical current flowing, which may in addition be responsible for the release of metal ions. Chronic exposure to mercury vapour may be responsible in some people for a range of symptoms such as headaches, memory loss, insomnia, tinnitus, gingivitis, and tremor.

An assessment carried out at the University of Kiel in Germany concluded that 'amalgam is a toxicologically unsuitable dentist filling material'. The Swedish dental association no longer recommends mercury fillings and the Swedish government is planning a phase-out of this substance.

Coffee filter paper

Coffee Filter Paper is bleached to make it white and look more acceptable. Bleach is a carcinogen.

Drugs

Drugs, which are chemicals, produced in factories. All drugs are poisons. Each drug is used for its poisonous effect on the body. There are no effects and side effects of drugs. There are only side effects. Doctors use a drug for one or another of its 'side effects' .The pain reduction of the common aspirin is a side effect or poison effect of aspirin. It has other side effects such as ulceration of the stomach lining causing bleeding.

Similarly anti-inflammatories are used for pain reduction and this is their 'effect' or 'side effect'. Between 15 000 to 20 000 Americans die every year from bleeding ulceration of the gastro- intestinal tract due to anti-inflammatories

Anti-inflammatories are perhaps the most dangerous of all medication in terms of the number of people dying from their use and the very high morbidity with over 100 000 people ending up in American hospitals because of bleeding.

Each drug is developed in such a way that the most useful 'side effect' e.g. pain reduction has a much higher profile that the more negative chemical reactions. In this way the pharmaceutical companies can claim that the benefits are much higher than the risks.

With pharmaceutical companies supporting most drug research programs and my own dubious attitude towards double blinds and the placebo response as indicated in another chapter, one needs to treat these results with some caution. Chronic long-term use of these chemicals to control symptoms is adding just another level of environmental poisons into the mix, which is also coming from other sources.

No one for example is doing research into what happens inside the body when drugs mix with the chlorine in the water, mercury vapour from the mouth, fluoride in the toothpaste, preservatives and colouring matter in the food, sulphur in the air, etc.

Plastic Wrap

Plastic is everywhere and even used for wrapping food. The best quality expensive wrapping may not leach toxic material into food but this is not what most people use. PVC plastic contains phthalates which have hormonal effects in the body while more modern plastic wrapping material is made from other chemicals which have not yet been fully investigated. New chemicals used in industry are generally allowed into the food chain before fully investigated for toxicity. Avoid using any material to wrap food or cook food in that does not contain an eco-friendly label.

Pesticides and Herbicides

There are about 630 different 'active ingredients' in pesticides worldwide. These ingredients are made up in thousands of different products on the market and are used to kill insects and fungus. They are highly toxic to the various living forms towards which they are directed. The labels on the container have warnings about there toxicity towards humans.

Many of the chemicals are now recognised carcinogens and have even been banned in various countries. With the movement of food across boundaries and the difficulty often of measuring all chemicals, the slow build-up of chemicals in animal tissue, water systems and the soil, there is an increasing amount of these chemicals filtering into the human body and often stored in the fatty tissue.

In the 10 years after Israel banned many toxic chemicals such as DDT and PCB the rate of breast cancer deaths declined sharply, with a 30% reduction in mortality for woman under 44 years of age. This is significant and should have made all countries stand up and take notice. Few have.

The WHO has recently warned people about the carcinogenicity of Roundup, perhaps the most used herbicide in the world today. This poison is sprayed indiscrimitely on farm land, in schools and children playgrounds to get rid of weeds, along road and pavements.

I have heard that farmers even spray Roundup on the potatoe crop plants to force an even die-off. Roundup does not just stay on the plants but gets into the soil and water supply and eventually into the blood of animals and humans, including babies.

Cigarettes and Cigarette Smoke

Research has clearly shown the relationship between smoking cigarettes, cancer and other diseases such as cardiovascular disease. Smoking is regarded as the biggest preventable cause of cancer accounting for 1 in 4 cancer deaths in many countries.

Tobacco was responsible for more than 100 million deaths worldwide in the 20th century. That's an enormous number and one would expect that these figures would influence people in their decision to stop or start smoking.

It has made a difference in many countries while in other countries young people still seem to be taking the risk. The problem is the addictive nature of nicotine found in tobacco. It takes less than 20 seconds for this chemical to reach the brain and is just as addictive as heroin and cocaine which are banned.

Many of the chemicals found in tobacco damage DNA and over time this DNA damage can no longer be repaired by the increasing dysfunction happening in other body systems due to the continued smoking, very often together with bad food choices of smokers plus other lifestyle mismanagements.

Industrial Chemicals

These include polychlorinated biphenols(PCBs), Perfluoro- octane sulfonate(PFOS) and perfluoro-octanoate (PFOA), Bisphenol A(BPA) and many others used in houshold items, clothing, carpets, furniture, personal care products and even plastic baby bottles, water bottles and lining of metal food cans. They all eventually end up in the water systems, soil and plants and found also in the blood of humans beings and animals.

Bisphenol A has been linked to breast[3] and prostate cancer[4]. In the USA it is now banned from use in baby bottles. Other bisphenols are replacing this one and already there is evidence of similar effects. This is the game that many companies play. So many new chemicals are appearing in the market place without adequate controls or research. It takes many years for any evidence of harm to appear. In the meantime children and adults are the 'rats' that are being testing for harm.

Phthalates is another group of chemicals known as plasticizers and found in cosmetics and personal care products, flexible plastic and vinyl toys, shower curtains, wall paper, food packaging, plastic wrap, wood finishes, detergents, adhesives, plastic plumbing pipes, lubricants, medical devices, building material and vinyl floors. Very

3   Grey J State of the evidence; The connection between breast cancer and the environment. 6th edition.Breast cancer Fund.2010

4   Prins GS Endocrine disruptors and prostate cancer risk. Endocr Relat Cancer 2008;15(3):649-656

difficult to escape exposure. The product has been linked to breast cancer[5] and listed as a carcinogen.

Parabens are commonly used in a range of products and I have noticed their presence in many 'health products' cosmetics as a preservative. They include methylparaben, propylparaben and butylparaben. They are recognised as carcinogenic but generally regarded as safe in the dose used.

The litany of poisonous substances in the environment is extensive and frightening. One must become concerned about what we are doing and allowing to be done to the environment. Governments, organizations and private individuals do need to take responsibility for poisoning the environment and the increase of cancer and the increasing chronic ill health that this is producing.

Many of the chemicals have not been adequately tested for human safety, banned chemicals such as DDT are still being used by farmers and despite regulations regarding the use of these chemicals farmers may still use these poisons indiscriminately.

Despite the fact that many of these chemicals and poisons are banned, restricted and unregistered in the USA, US manufacturers are still allowed to produce and export these substances mainly to 3rd world countries. Fruit and vegetables are then imported back into the USA. Only about half of the pesticides in use can be identified by current testing methods.

Many of these chemicals are called xenobiotics, hormone disruptors or estrogen mimics because they can interfere with the hormonal balance in females as well as males and may be an important factor for the increasing infertility occuring today.

Petrochemical compounds may be found in general consumer products such as creams, lotions, soaps, shampoos, perfumes, hair sprays and room deodorizers. Such compounds often have chemical structures similar to estrogen and indeed act like estrogen.

Other sources of xenoestrogens include car exhaust, petrochemically derived pesticides, herbicides, and fungicides,

5   Lopez-Carillo L et al . Exposure to phthalates and
     breast cancer risk in northen mexico. Environ Health
     perspect 2010; 118(4):539-544

solvents and adhesives such as those found in nail polish, paint removers, and glues, dry-cleaning chemicals, practically all plastics, industrial waste such as PCBs and dioxins, synthetic estrogens from urine of women taking HRT and birth control pills that are flushed down the toilet and eventually find their way into the food chain and back into the body.

They are fat soluble and non-biodegradable industrial solvents. A common source of industrial xenoestrogens often overlooked is a family of chemicals called solvents. These chemicals enter the body through the skin, and accumulate quickly in the lipid-rich tissues such as myelin (nerve sheath) and adipose (fat).

Some common organic solvents include alcohol like methanol, aldehydes like acetaldehyde, glycol like ethylene glycol, and ketones like acetone. They are commonly found in cosmetics, fingernail polish and fingernail polish remover, glues, paints, varnishes, and other types of finishes, cleaning products, carpet, fiberboard, and processed woods. Pesticides and herbicides such as lawn and garden sprays, indoor insect sprays are also sources of minute amounts of xenoestrogens. While the amount may be small in each, the additive effect from years of chronic exposure can lead to estrogen dominance.

Discussion

We have become dull minded by the absolute deluge of chemicals in the environment and the damage caused often seems like a distant dream, much like climate change which for many people does not changed their immediate lives. Something that will happen but not in my life time!

Unfortunately there is a major cover up by industry and even governments. This cover up is a somewhat understandible. Once an industry gets going and becomes as powerful as the chemical industry, cigarette industry, petro-chemical industry, they cannot just be replaced with alternative sources that may be cheaper, more healthy and require different technology without causes a major loss of jobs to thousands if not millions of people around the world. So we keep hearing the following reasons for not shifting the goal posts:

- The benefits are worth the risk.

- There is not enough scientific evidence.

- We are already doing what is required to warn people and reduce smoking, emissions, dangers of side effects.

- There are no better alternatives.

- The problem is really not as serious as everyone suggests.

There are of course very often better alternative or at least other choices that could work, but the effort, money and time involved is too much for governments and the lay public to even contemplate.

At what point does the risk no longer seem justfied?

That is a really interesting question that has often troubled me when a patients sits in front of me and the question of chemotherapy for cancer comes up. We live in a world of complexity when prediction of human life span in the face of serious disease is as difficult to define as weather prediction.

We have our statistics to help us but in dealing with individual cases it is often experience which helps us more but can just as often let us down. Governments and academics go on averages and statistics where answers seem clear over time, whereas the individual is less interested in the statistics but wants to know about his own chances of recovery. Here is the 'grey area' again when suddenly face to face with the real world.

There is also the question of biochemical individuality. This is the very unique particular biochemical functionality (based on genetic code) that all of us have and often means that the need for a particular nutrient for example may be much more than another person. Normal for that person falls outside the common normal. This will therefore mean that assessing risk vs benefit will have to take into account the person's unique profile, background and genetics.

Not enough scientific evidence

This is another problem area. How much science is enough science. Can one trust scientific research driven by the very companies that are selling the product and the regulatory bodies that are even funded by these same companies.

- Enormous bias by pharmaceutical companies

- Negative studies not published

- Large payouts to doctors and laboratories for results that support the use of drugs.

- Use of ghost writters who actually was not involved directly in the study.

The way regulatory bodies, officials and Big Pharma manage to delay regulations when it seems obvious that the medication could be harmful and even seriously harmful is to say that there 'is not enough scientific evidence'. When peoples lives are at stake then when does enough evidence become enough.

Regulators, government officials and specialists have a very different outlook on the above question than the public and others who are concerned about public health. Iatrogenic disease (doctor induced ill health) which I have discussed in other chapters is the 3rd or 4th most common cause of ill health and death .

Every regulator knows this but from the viewpoint they have the benefits are worth the risk. That is, the fact that people die means that others may live and have a better life. People die in war but the government in power believes that the benefits are worth the risk and fact that thousands of young men and women are going to die. It is just the nature of things.

Doing all that is required to save peoples lives

- Obesity is pandemic around the world in rich first world counteries and 3rd world country's

- If something like marijuana can be banned and this does not have nearly the level of side effect of cigarettes then why does every country around the world allow cigarettes on sale?

No better alternatives!

What this usually means is that the money train is moving in a particular direction that works for a lot of people in power. Alternatives are everywhere. We have just converted our regular pool using chlorine into a biologically friendly pond by creating a wet land with plants .

It has taken a while to get the algae under control during the hot summer months but using an ultraviolet light there is now good control. No more chlorine and other chemicals to pollute. All our cleaning solutions in the kitchen are biologically friendly. They will be more expensive until more people use them so that the price can drop.

The public needs to take some responsibility for the pollution and shift the money trail towards non-polluting items and stamp their feet when necessary. The chemical residue left after washing utensils by hand or dishwasher, on our clothes which we wear after washing with chemicals can all get absorbed into the body and add to the total load of carcinogens, xenoestrogens and antibiotics.

So we come in the end to the sad truth. Govenments won't and probably cannot make real changes regarding pollution control because of the financial cost involved. Human beings are dispensable. We are part of the business model whose bottom line is financial and not health. This attitude will only shift if people rise up and demand such a change. So become the change you want by first making changes in your own home.

The following are some guidelines:

- Water filters essential. Remember also to place a water filter in your shower.

- Grow your own organic vegetables or buy local at the farmers markets.

- Buy only raw milk if available

- Eat only pasture raised animal meat or venison.

- Avoid junk foods and processed foods

- Avoid refined oils and only used cold pressed oils.

- Avoid margarines

- No Smoking

- While 1-2 glasses of red wine are usually permitted, be carefully of doing this daily as alcohol is a toxin to the liver.

- Use biodegradable cleaning solutions in your kitchen and house generally.

- Change your chlorinated pool to a biologically active pool.

- Solar heaters

The environment is serious toxic and poisonous to healthy living. Everywhere these pollutants are creeping into our body systems. The school playground your children run around, often barefoot is sprayed with Roundup and other carcinogenic chemicals to control the weeds.

If the school is close to a farm then on a windy day those chemicals used by the farmer are drifting into the classroom. Remember that passive smoking is almost as dangerous as the real thing. The most common pollutants in water are disinfection byproducts, nitrate, and arsenic.

Nitrates enter the drinking water from fertilizer runoff, leaching of septic tanks, and erosion of natural deposits and a range of industrial sources and mining contamination. The municipalities in many towns spray the trees for mildew and the walkaway with weed killers. Not to mention of course the fact that pollutants are also falling out of the sky from thousands of airoplanes constantly in the air. Winds carry pollutants all over the world so that even in places like the North and South Pole the breast milk of mothers contain pollutants that are not from local use.

It is important to keep in mind one message of this book and that is while it is true that any single chemical or pollutant can cause harm above a certain dose in a susceptible person, what we are generally concerned about is the synergy effect, the accumulated effect of a mass of pollutants in small doses and how this works itself out in any individual.

Smoking becomes seriously more toxic when other pollutants are also present. Lead and mercury even in small doses when present in infants who have not yet developed a strong, robust immune system can cause serious harm. The same would apply to passive smoke from their smoking parents which hangs around in the air for many hours.

Toxins must be removed by the main organ of detoxification which is the liver. With the increasing amounts of children and people developing fatty livers from poor diets, the ability to detox these pollutants becomes more difficult.

So it is important to keep in mind that when government agencies and industry points to scientific studies to show that these pollutants are actually not as serious as many people make it out to be, a great deal of the time they are referring to research on animals where single chemicals are tested or studies where the time frame is too short to make the kind of conclusions that are generally made from these studies.

No one wants to turn the present system on its head. Imagine research suggesting that chlorine, which is a form of bleach is actually harmful to human beings. One would almost immediately see the industry coming up with research which pointed to the weakness in the science, that the scientists involved were biased and lastly that still more science was needed.

Individuals are finally left on their own to make these decisions. Make a good decision that includes the welfare of those close to you and the people you come in contact with.

Chapter 11

She had tried unsuccessfully to commit suicide on three different occassions. Each time she was confronted by parents that were horrified but tried not to show it, friends that could not understand, colleagues at work that felt sorry for her, but when at last she was diagnosed with cancer she confided in me how she could die peacefully now with everyone feeling so much more compassionate towards her, her parents genuinely surrounding her with the kind of love she craved and everyone really supportive.

She obviously refused chemotherapy and was happy that surgery was not possible. She had a radiance of peace and even joy until she died very peacefully.

The Meaning of Illness

There are many levels upon which an understanding of illness can be investigated. Consider a young man of 29 years old who complains for the first time of developing an eczema of his hands. He has been working in the same factory for 5 years and nothing has changed in his work situation over those years.

The first doctor he goes to makes a diagnosis of contact dermatitis i.e. an allergic rash due to contact with a chemical agent at work and gives him cortisone cream. The rash clears up but he notices that each time he stops using the cream the rash appears again. He returns to the doctor who takes a more careful history and gives him some suggestions about finding out what it is in his workplace that has caused the allergy.

The man is more careful this time, trying to notice what in his environment could be a causative factor and avoiding handling anything which may aggravate the rash. In the meantime he continues to use the cortisone cream noticing again that the cream is only symptomatic. The problem however continues and he is a little disconcerted to notice one morning that there is a small patch of eczema on his chest which is irritating and itchy.

He goes to a dermatologist for a second opinion and leaves with a prescription for a stronger cortisone based cream and cortisone injection. The injection is long acting and he is symptom-free for more than a month. Just when he is beginning to forget about the rash one morning he wakes up again with an itch on his chest, arms and back and too his horror there is now a spreading rash all over his upper body.

Having spoken to colleagues at work he begins to realise that the conventional route usually means more cortisone creams and injections and not much chance of real recovery. A second opinion is called for and perhaps alternative therapies should be considered. He finds out the name of a holistic doctor and makes an appointment. This time he goes a little wiser and has some pertinent questions to ask:

- If this is a contact dermatitis, then why now after five years in the same work environment?

- Why me?

- Could stress play a role?

- Would diet make a difference?

- Could it be hereditary and appear at this age?

- Can it be cured?

- Why eczema?

- Is there a cure?

These are obviously important questions and generally do not get addressed by conventional doctors who find it more convenient to prescribe cortisone creams and use injections than spending more time with the patient. Many patients in addition really want a quick fix and hope that the cortisone prescription will be the quick answer.

This patient's questions do begin to address the complexity of the problem. We have discussed the multiplicity of causes in other chapters and again here we can see that in all probability a number of factors have come together to initiated the patient's condition.

In fact the holistic doctor discusses diet management in detail and suggests an elimination diet in which the patient eliminates all colouring matter, preservatives, milk, wheat and gluten products, stops using all processed foods and eliminates sugar and sugar based products such as soda drinks, cakes, doughnuts, ice-cream etc. The simplicity and discipline required for such a diet in itself is helpful and is a first step in a holistic management of allergy problems.

What about stress and why me? Here we come to the crux of this chapter so we need to spend more time in trying to understand the real complexity and the depth of co-operation and trust required between the doctor and patient. Many patients are aware of the relationship between their physical condition and stress. They usually notice that when they are stressed their physical symptoms and signs seem to become worse. It usually does not surprise them although they are often surprised if a doctor should suggest that stress is the cause of a condition such as eczema.

We have discussed in previous chapters the relationship between mind and body. Learning to drive a motorcar has everything to do with the relationship between mind and body so there should be no surprise that mind can influence body.

How is mind and stress responsible for a condition such as eczema? If a person is angry, then one can usually see on their face and the general body language gives clues to the emotion that that person is having. The person may try and hide their emotion but even then the signs of stress are still visible in the eyes and body language.

What happens to the emotion when not expressed outwardly? Certainly the body still feels the emotion even when it is unexpressed outwards. It is this 'feeling' which is important in the way a disease may develop.

The relationship between mind and body has been very well investigated in what is referred to as 'psychosomatic medicine'.

When a person is angry and this is expressed outwardly there are obvious characteristics, which allow most of us to identify the emotion as anger. The facial expressions, the angry look in the eyes, the way the arms and body move all indicate the anger that the person feels.

In a similar way any anger that is suppressed will have a corresponding 'energetic signature tune'. By this I mean that the specific tension and the energetic/physiological pattern which it initiates within the body has a characteristic that corresponds to that particular hidden emotion.

Each person's anger is not exactly the same as another's, especially when there is an attempt at suppression. Then it is often mixed with resentment, frustration, bitterness, indignation, jealousy, wounded pride, feeling hurt, vengefulness etc., each aspect putting its own particular stamp on the 'energetic/physiological signature tune'.

Let me explain the idea of the 'energetic/physiological signature tune', which helps me to understand the relationship between mind and body and the development of ill health. Each emotion such as anxiety, anger, resentment etc. has its own particular character, which seems to start as a thought and become an emotion.

Neither the thought nor the emotion can be measured by science but there is a clear recognition of the different character of one emotion and another. We are often less aware of the subtleties between our various emotional states but there is a whole spectrum of variation in each of the various emotional experiences.

Emotions are also not simple but have a mix of a range of different reactions all happening at the same time. For example, anger and resentment may be swirling together in the same person. A feeling of being a victim, may be accompanied by a sense of hopelessness, fear, heaviness, dull minded.

Every one of these feelings and emotions casts it own energetic colour over the whole biochemical profile of that person, causing hormonal shifts, immune system disturbances, gastro-intestinal changes, stomach acid depression or increase, heart rate rhythm effects, sympathetic and parasympathetic pressures etc.

No Part of the Body Chemistry and Function Remains Untouched by our Feeling / emotional Self

Yet there is very little science to thinking and emotions. I do need however to mention that many scientists would point to the fact that one can record electromagnetic and other measurable changes in brain activity today with sensitive instruments. It is not at all clear that these recordings of brain activity are actually the emotion or reflecting the effect of emotions on the brain structures. Which came first!

Are human beings electromagnetic/physiological beings which can be measured or is this the expression of something much deeper and more subtle which cannot be measured.

This becomes important is the question of 'meaning'. It is highly unlikey that chemicals in the body are interested in meaning. The same would apply to electromagnetic fields. Animals and plants don't seem to be interested in meaning either. So the whole question of 'meaning' is a particular human condition and takes us deeper into the fabric of what it means to be human.

It seems that we perhaps give too much value to what can be measured and then downgrade life in general and human life in particular to mechanism which can be manipulated because they can be measured and at the same time stop looking for other qualities outside measurement because they don't fit into our paradigm.

If meaning is important to human beings then can shifting the meaning towards ill health have an effect on the outcome of management?

But back to the signature tune.

That signature tune of a stressful emotion, if it is suppressed, goes on playing in the subconscious and will eventually emerge as a symptom within the body. Where it emerges, its severity and its particular character will depend on the energy and type of the emotion suppressed.

Each particular subconsciously suppressed emotion has its own particular energetic signature tune and may eventually express itself within the body as ill health. The principle is not different to my thought for my hand to go up ending with my hand going up or my emotion of anger showing itself up as an expression on my face.

The way this subconscious signature tune eventually expresses itself will have the hallmark and signature of its underlying stressful factors. We all know what anger, depression, happiness and joy for example looks like when expressed outwardly. It is surprising how often one has the feeling that the illness is saying something, that it is talking to us about the person, about his needs, her frustrations, deep seated wishes unfulfilled.

Have you noticed how being with an ill person seems to call up within you the question 'why are you really ill and the recognition that there is something you are trying to say'? The language of metaphor and bodily symptoms and signs is well described in many books and the English language has many expressions indicating the underlying emotional conflict for bodily symptoms. Here are some examples:

- Shoulder pain = carrying burdens, your own and other peoples' problems.

- Stiff neck = stubbornness

- Indigestion = not digesting life properly

- Blindness = not wanting to see

- Deafness = not wanting to hear

- Stomach ulcer = eating oneself up about an issue

- Eczema = irritation and oversensitive

- Hay fever = overreacting to someone and trying to blow them away

- Back problems = lack of support in one's life

- Elbow pain = wanting to elbow someone out of the way

- Heel pain or spur = sticking one heels in i.e. not wanting to move.

- Cystitis = pissed off with someone

- Throat problems = blocked expression

- Hands = difficulty in handling life

- Cancer = self destructive thoughts and emotions

- Insomnia = fear of letting go

- Nail biting = frustration

- Stuttering = insecurity

- Vomiting = rejection of ideas

- Feet problems = something you cannot stand

- Skin cancer = something or someone close getting under one's skin

- Food allergy = cannot stomach something

All this may seem very simplistic yet it is surprising how often an enquiry along these lines will in fact reveal an underlying emotional conflict which has been simmering below the surface. Try to actually feel each emotion and see the connection to the physical disease.

As indicated in previous chapters there are no single causes to an illness and this multiplicity of causes does make the expression of the ill health quite complex yet I am always surprised how in a willing patient the underlying expression of the illness will reveal its hidden message of emotional conflict when questioned.

I am surprised how often people are really even thankful when I, the doctor, ask them what they think the meaning of the illness is to them. It seems that they are just waiting for this question because when asked then suddenly the story that needs to be connected to the ill health emerges.

Feel the emotion and how it connects to the body. Look at the body and understand the message.

The body language often expresses the inner concerns of the person much more effectively and truthfully than the words the person is using.

A lady of 35 years of age came to see me for infertility. On testing it emerged that her father had often expressed his dismay with her and that she would never succeed in anything. Her deep-seated fear was that she would not be able to cope with the pregnancy and would not be able to look after the baby. She was actually afraid of becoming pregnant and yet had been running around from one doctor to another insisting that she wanted to fall pregnant and had allowed herself to go through a great deal of expensive investigations and treatment.

Another patient came for an overweight problem. On questioning it became apparent that there was a deep resistance to losing weight. Her overweight problem was hiding a deep rejection of herself as a woman. Obviously her overweight was reflecting her fear of being noticed by men and was something she could hide behind yet for years she followed one diet after another in order to loose weight without any success.

There are different levels of understanding that one may enter into in trying to understand the meaning of ill health. I remember a book given to me as a present when I was still at school. It contained anatomical pictures of the body in which one could peel back one page after the other revealing deeper and deeper layers, from the skin surface, muscle layer then the organs to the bones.

How deep do you want to go?

So it is with the meaning of a person's symptoms and signs. At the most superficial level the symptoms and signs represent some underlying physical problem, for example painful muscle spasm in the back may be due to a disc protruding causing muscle spasm to prevent movement.

On a deeper level the back represents support systems and may indicated emotional frustration at not being supported by a spouse. On a still deeper level the back problem may indicate a psycho-spiritual conflict in not feeling supported by spirit or God.. Some healers may even see in the back problem some karmic and past lives issues that need to be dealt with.

The human being is not just a physical body but has enfolded within that body other 'bodies' each one more subtle than the other and yet each body reflecting something of the other all the way through into the physical. Chapter 13 'The human body revisited' describes these energy fields and their relationship to the physical body. The symptoms and signs in the physical body are therefore the visible reflection of the deeper invisible layers and are full of meaning.

How deep each person wants to go in discovering the meaning of their ill health is again full of meaning. Many people prefer to follow the conventional medical model and ascribe the underlying cause of their ill health to micro-organism, past injuries, cigarette smoking or excessive alcohol consumption. Others may begin to enquire around the reasons why they are involved in self destructive behaviours, or whether the accident was really an accident or was part of a much bigger story or whether the particular condition they were suffering from was indeed a message to them from their higher self.

I am using words freely and metaphorically. Choose a meaning that comes up for you but choose a meaning that enriches. Notice how meaning that enriches also results in 'feeling' better as apposed to meaning that dissipates energy. Notice that something in you is choosing the meaning and that one has the ability to change the story and create a different meaning.

Changing a person's story and the meaning of the illness is very much part of my practice of medicine. I sometimes think that it is the most important part of my consultation. It really is not difficult to become aware of the dramatic shift in the way the body responds and the feelings one has within the body with a change in the story line and the meaning that comes with it.

Change the Story and Change the Body Responses

My experience is that most, if not all, illnesses are not hapharzard occurences and that the underlying causes and meaning can become a life long journey of self discovery. I do recognise that this is a particular viewpoint which may challenge many colleagues and others reading this far.

I am extending myself beyond conventional medical science and into a world that most people and patients recognise and live. Nevertheless I am always surprised to hear very conventional and reductionistic and materialistic scientists use words in normal conversation such as feeling, I think, I know, bliss, what a joy, my grandchild makes me feel young again, I love walking in nature, I had an intuitive moment etc. These are normal experiences of human beings that cannot be measured, are subjective, that carry a message that others can still understand, that can be given 'degrees' of power and can cause others to respond or react.

We are subjective beings and this 'reality' cannot be dismissed by an objective science looking for causes only within its scope of reference.

As a doctor I need to be open and responsive to the patient's subjective world. It is too complex for me to really understand any more than I can understand fully my own subjective space and why I often react in a negative way to a particular stimulus. As we relate to each other within the space we are sharing, as I listen carefully to the patient's story and help the patient develop a map within which he or she can find a place to rest and look around, a level of control begins to emerge. It is something like spending a whole day in a city that you have never been to before and then coming home and looking at a map of the city and suddenly all the places you visited begin to have an order. The next day when visiting the city all the places have a context and one can now go a little deeper into the city's heart.

Meaning is Everything!

Finding meaning in an illness gives that illness a depth to it that was not there before. The illness can also take one really deep into oneself especially when it does not just dissapear. The back pain moves from being caused by an injury only, to why do I feel lacking in support, to a childhood incidence of getting lost and not finding parents to support one, to the very essence of understanding the nature of fear and then even deeper to acknowledging the fear of death itself where all support seems to dissapear.

The depth one goes is unique to each person. There is no right or wrong way but only the way one chooses which is the only way you can go because that is the choice you have made. Illness itself is not 'wrong' unless you make it wrong . The flow of life is not 'wrong' either unless you see it in a negative way.

We are constantly choosing the way we want to see 'reality'. Illness to my way of thinking is always an attempt at correcting a disharmony that has arisen on some deeper level . It is the way the unconscious drama happening below the surface of the conscious mind slowly or even rapidly rises to the surface.

The 'war' against cancer and in fact the attitude against all disease by the medical profession has created the idea of a battle, something bad and destructive about disease. Disease must be got rid of as soon as possible!

I am pointing to something very different here, of seeing ill health as an opportunity to change ones life, to find deeper meaning and raise one's consciousness towards a deepening of love and compassion for self and others. Right attitude towards illness, a real respect for the body and the way it is handling itself, finding a good story that makes sense to oneself will go a long way to stimulating healing chemicals in the body and turning around ill health.

Ill Health is an Opportunity to Discover the Meaning and Even Direction of One's Life Journey

So while finding meaning to ill health is certainly not part of the medical curriculum, it is nevertheless a powerful healing tool that can not only change the thinking-emotional patterns but also effect real changes in the physical body. Psychologists in the field of 'psychoneuroimmunology' have shown that the state of the mind can affects the health of the body particularly the immune system.

A massive review[1] body of nearly 300 studies on stress and health showed that stress of any signficant duration, from a few days to a few months or years, as happens in real life, affected immunity, which went downhill.

1   Segerstrom SC & Miller GE 2004. Psycho- logical
     stress and the human Immune System. A
     Meta-Analysis study of 30 years of inquiry.
     Psychological Bulletin. 130.4.

It is good to keep in mind that stress starts in the thinking mind which works its way into our emotional responses which then spreads through the physiological system. The 'meaning' that we give to life, our ill health, our work situation, to politics, to our relationships, to our body , to our journey – all of that has an effect 'all the way down' into every cell of the body either supporting health or obstructing the flow.

Chapter 12

She clearly was into fitness. It's easy to tell. She was carrying a bottle of water, still in her gym clothes and carried herself upright and yet her facial expression was confused and brows furrowed in deep concentration.

'If I am so fit doctor,' she said 'how come I don't feel well?'

She was one of those that Integrative doctors call the 'walking ill'. They are everywhere, not really understanding why despite going to the gym 2 or even 3 times per week, cutting down on junk food and having stopped smoking and drinking too much alcohol are still worried about their health.

All the tests doctors have done come back normal suggesting that there is no disease present in their body.

'So what is wrong with me doctor? Is it all in my mind?'

Health and Harmony

What is health and how do we know when we are healthy? These are not questions that can be easily answered. I have known individuals who have walked out of a specialists rooms having just passed through the usual ECG and other common tests with flying colours and suffered a heart attack in the lift on the way out of the building.

Many cancer patients have been extremely well until on routine examination a lump is diagnosed which turns out to be malignant. Thousands upon thousands of people without any symptoms and who regard themselves as normal and healthy are diagnosed every day with high blood pressure, high cholesterol, early diabetes, abnormal pap smears, cancers, enlarged prostates, nodules on thyroids and other medical conditions and yet would of regarded themselves as healthy. Modern medicine has made possible the detection of a whole range of diseases, which until fairly recently would have gone undetected.

Is a person who feels well and regards himself in good health indeed healthy if he has an underlying high blood pressure, increased cholesterol or even a hidden cancer? How are we to incorporate ideas of psychological health? Is this separate from health of the physical body? If a person is depressed, but physically healthy, is such a person to be regarded as healthy? Is psychological health or physical health more important?

We can begin to see how complicated this issue is and that no simple answer is possible. Collins dictionary defines health as physical and mental well-being; freedom from disease. As indicated above physical and mental well-being does not mean that the person is however free of disease. It is possible of course that as our means of detecting the earlier stages of disease becomes more sensitive, that more and more people will be labelled as ill without having any symptoms and signs.

Already today many thousands of "healthy" individuals are taking expensive medication for high blood pressure long before it produces any obvious symptoms. This medication must be taken for the rest of that person's life and may produce mild to severe and even life threatening ill health. The benefits of taking the medication are regarded as better than the risks of not taking the medication. I will be looking at the issue of drugs in another chapter but let us for the moment concentrate on the issue of health.

Can one be healthy and sick at the same time?

No one comes into the world perfect. Each individual has a host of physical and mental potential Achilles heels. No motor car comes out of the factory perfect, but it does not break down immediately. It requires many other factors, which put pressure on the system as a whole before in time something becomes obvious that the machine is not functioning as it should. The arrow of breakdown the problem takes will depend on the totality of all the pressures in the system.

Factory problem - - - > Breakdown

No machine comes out of the factory perfect and one could say therefore that from the moment it moves out of the factory it is moving towards its breakdown point. Similarly with the human being. No one comes out of the factory perfect. Genetic factors are more or less important in any person's life so that from the moment of birth one is moving towards the breakdown point aided by many other stress factors. The final breakdown is of course death. These points will be examined in other chapters.

The point is then that no one can really claim to be perfectly healthy. All that can be stated is that the person feels in good health physically and mentally or does not.

The next step would be the examination and investigations. It is at this point that the problem starts in trying to define health. Examination and investigation may be useful, confusing or even dangerous. The problem is not the obvious case of disease, but the 'borderline and unusual' , the false positives and false negatives, the mind-body connection, the fear and worry generated by even the thought of ill health and many doctors attitudes which are not helpful and healing. Large numbers of people fit into this category. Medical doctors often encourage yearly checkups, but this could be dangerous to your health. What is your individual normal and can early cancer and/or other diseases disappear before they cause a problem.

Medical routine examinations and investigations can be dangerous to one's health.

Medical science is already pointing to the fact that finding earlier cancers such as early stage prostate cancer or early stage ductal cell cancers of the breast, thyroid cancers and even some lung cancers should perhaps not even be labelled as cancers because many or even most of them don't ever require treatment.

Calling them cancers immediately moves the person in the direction of 'cancer therapy' and the consequences that may go with it in terms of anxiety, side effects of treatment and the long term follow up and expense with more investigations than are often required. Apart from the suffering many relatively healthy people die along the way as a result of all the investigations .

In an article entitled 'Addressing over-diagnosis and overtreatment in cancer: a prescription for change' published in the prestigious peer reviewed journal Lancet Oncology, a group of medical professors suggest a change in naming many of these early cancers and rather call them 'indolent lesions' of epithelial origin. This is a brave and innovative statement. They suggest that these lesions are very low risk and that repeated and early screening is just bringing these early lesions to the attention of doctors.

'Screening guidelines should be revised to lower the chance of detection of minimal risk indolent lesions and inconsequential cancers with the same energy traditionally used to increase the sensitivity of screening tests.'[1]

1   Lancet Oncol 2014 May

Even modern sophisticated examinations do not resolve the problem of false positives and negatives but often just increase the confusion. A member of the family had a CT scan for a very painful arm for many months. The report suggested fluid within the muscle and a tear in the capsule of the shoulder. Surgery was decided as the only chance in view of the above. The surgery found no such problem but just wear and tear in the shoulder joint.

The 'normal' that doctors quote are statistical normals only. They are averages and not your individual normal. The body is enormously complex and always compensating for any stress in one part of the system by attempting to make a correction in another part.

We don't know the cause of high blood pressure, but it could be a correcting factor in order to maintain a balance in the system as a whole. The person with high blood pressure is generally without any symptoms and signs. Biochemical results also have a great deal of variation between individuals and even of the same individual when measured over time. For this reason doctors generally like to retest abnormal results not only because of laboratory errors, but also because of variation of body functions and changes in the level of blood tests.

No two individuals have exactly the same biochemical profile and the response to any stimuli will create a movement of change that will also reflect this unique and individual variation. Human beings are characterised more by their individuality and variability than by what they have in common.

Each individual has a unique characteristic fingerprint as well as other characteristics which are different, such as blood groups, immunoglobulins, antibodies, genetic make-up, etc. Each one of these differences will influence the response of the person to create an individual complex of symptoms and signs.

Each individual has a range of unique characteristics which apply all the way down to biochemistry and energy.

Normal values are statistical values only. Many of these normal values accepted in general by doctors throughout the world may be dated, belonging to ethnic groups from another country and are always arbitrary values decided upon by specialist groups of doctors from limited number of people.

There are huge profits to be made by pharmaceutical companies if the normal value for the blood pressure is set at a lower level. A 5-point difference only could boost profits for anti-hypertensives by many millions of dollars. The same situation applies to whatever decision is made regarding the 'normal' cholesterol blood level.

The pharmaceutical companies that have most to gain from the sale of anti-cholesterol drugs finance most of the research. The lower the normal values are pegged, the more people become labelled as ill with high cholesterol levels despite the fact that these individuals may feel completely healthy, they now have a label of ill health. Do normal values change over decades or centuries? Is there a different normal for ethnic groups or on different continents? In the life history of each person, is there a change in the profile of normal?

The more investigations one has the more likely the chances of finding an abnormality and being labelled with a disease diagnosis.

Normal or abnormal based on biochemistry are statistical normal only based on a relatively small number of individuals

These questions have not been seriously addressed so that, once again, one can begin to recognize the real problem in deciding what is normal for that individual and at what point can one clearly state that the condition is now abnormal and diseased.

A person can also feel seriously ill and yet have no symptoms and signs of disease.

In trying to define health therefore the best one can do is perhaps to state the obvious i.e. a person can only be regarded as relatively healthy if that person feels in general healthy; physically, emotionally and mentally; and if a general routine examination by a competent doctor reveals no evidence of disease.

Further investigation should only be undertaken if there is a good indication and not routinely as is the practice at the moment. An enormous amount of routine investigations are really for medico-legal reasons and not for the health of the person. These investigations include PSA tests for prostate cancer, mammograms for breast cancer and biopsies for prostate and thyroid cancers .

These latter tests must be decided on an individual basis. Some of them would be regarded as essential for anyone over 50 years of age. Many doctors would regard these tests as essential before giving the individual a clean bill of health. The truth however is that most of the doctors who insist that these tests are essential do not perform these tests on themselves.

Why is this so? The reasons are complex and generally reflect the doctor's fears, and often overwork with insufficient time to look after his own health. Apart from suffering the very same fears as their patients, doctors also understand the problems. False positives and false negatives are serious issues and many tests are not easy to interpret. Consider the following examples:

A patient has back pain and a narrow disc space is seen on   X-ray. Is this the cause of his pain? Narrowed disc spaces are common findings especially in the elderly and the vast majority of people do not have any pain from this. The public regard ECGs as important in the diagnosis of heart disease, yet even stress ECGs are considered as less than 40% accurate and some reports suggest that they may be even useless in predicting heart disease. Diagnosis from tests is dependent on training and experience of specialists and this can vary and account for many of the false positives and negatives. An example is the common Pap smear.

This test is dependent on good technique, the use of the right tools and taking the specimen from the correct anatomical position. This may seem straight forward to any layperson, but in fact anatomy varies enormously and the view of the cervix may not be clear. The scrapings are smeared onto a glass slide and in the process the cells may be so damaged as to suggest abnormalities. The cells may be further damaged on the way to the laboratory.

False positives are as fraught with risk as false negatives. A false positive will lead to anxiety and stress on the person concerned. Further tests are instituted. Each test is more expensive than the previous one and more and more specialists become involved. With the great variation and uniqueness of each individual the problem does not always become clearer the more tests are done and the more specialists are consulted. The case may seem to be more serious than initially thought so that surgery is even contemplated to resolve the problem. Surgery has risks attached and so one problem leads to another.

I have painted the negative side of this process. There is also the positive side in which a routine Pap smear picks up a very early carcinoma. Most doctors, it seems, and also their patients are afraid. Afraid of false positives, false negatives and even afraid that maybe there may be something there which requires further treatment. Each person in the end must deal with his or her own destiny. I don't believe that the condition of health and disease can be dealt with in a hypothetical way as if health is a condition separate from disease and that there is a clear distinction between the two.

Health and disease are like seasons. They flow into each other. Disease draws out of health a response and health even needs disease for its well being just as a sportsman needs competition for his progress. The best stimulus for the immune system is a viral infection and it is possible that many of the viral infections in children are necessary to strengthen the immune response over time and even part of the evolutionary cycle required for good health.

Immune system health may depend on recurrent childhood viral infections

I will deal with this issue in other chapters, but suffice to say here that health and disease should be approached in a much more dynamic way. One needs to recognize that even when a person regards himself as ill, he is still more healthy than ill. The individuals lungs are still absorbing oxygen, the food eaten is still being digested and nourishment is still flowing to every cell. Poisons are constantly being removed and the acid / alkaline balance of the blood and temperature are generally still being maintained within normal levels. When a person is much more ill than healthy then we can regard such a person as almost dead or terminal. An ill person is therefore much more healthy than ill. It is only that the healthy part does not make a noise.

Even when ill, the system is more healthy overall than it is ill.

This is somewhat akin to a hall full of people where a few are making a noise and it seems as if everyone is noisy. The fact is that only a handful of people are making all the noise and the majority are just sitting still watching the show. Nevertheless the noisy few can totally disrupt the show and prevent the others from enjoying themselves. A seriously painful toe can affect you not only emotionally and mentally but the process includes a metabolic inflammatory shift in the toe which pushes out inflammatory chemicals affecting the whole body causing tiredness, foggy thinking and even depression.

If we try to review this chapter on trying to define health then one must admit that disease and even death for that matter are constant companions of health. No one is perfectly healthy and therefore everyone is a little ill. This is not unhealthy in itself despite the fact that people die from ill health and disease. What is important however is that we find ways to support the system in its attempts to heal itself and to improve health rather than focus too much attention on the ill health. This is an important consideration and will be covered in later chapters. In a world as polluted as it is today, with stress levels as high as they are everywhere, with food choices that are not always the best options, we no longer can leave it to chance and the body's own devices in order to function optimally.

Health and ill health are flowing systems at work. Supporting health will decrease ill health.

If freedom of symptoms and signs is no criteria of health then should we all be going for more and more tests to try to identify the ill health that we have as soon as possible? As indicated above, even here there are serious problems. False positives and false negatives and the danger of investigations cannot be dismissed easily. Let me illustrate this problem with some case histories.

A man of 65 years has a routine prostate enzyme study (PSA). He has had this before on at least three occasions and they have always been normal. This time however the result is considerably above normal. He does have a large prostate, but no evidence suggesting cancer. Benign prostatic enlargement had been diagnosed on previous occasions. His GP sends him to a specialist who feels a little unsure now about the prostate and suggests a biopsy.

A biopsy is an invasive procedure in which a number of punctures are made through the capsule of the prostate in order to obtain biopsies from different parts of the prostate. All these biopsies are reported as showing only inflammatory cells and he is given antibiotics for one month. His urine is now bloody from the biopsy and he continues to have pain for some months.

The pain, which he never had before, together with the bloody urine has created a certain phobia and fear of cancer. He no longer is sure that the doctors have told him the whole truth and he worries about cancer. The prostate enzymes returned to normal soon after the biopsy. There is also the theoretical risk that if cancer is present in the prostate, a needle biopsy by piercing the capsule of the prostate may contribute to spreading the cancer outside the capsule.

A gentleman has had a mole on his back for almost 10 years. His doctor has suggested on many occasions that he is unhappy with the mole and should have it removed. Eventually the man challenges the doctor to remove the mole, which he does in his rooms. The mole is malignant and a specialist performs a more extensive removal of tissue. Within days of this latter operation, the man begins to complain of pain around his chest. He has never had pain or any symptoms before. 15 months later he still has severe pain, which is not controlled very well by pain pills.

All doctors have cases like this and for this reason they are often very hesitant to become involved themselves with investigations. Each person in the end must take responsibility for his or her own life. I don't believe there is a right or wrong way. Each person lives out his or her own destiny. It is a game of chance because no matter what the statistics show, your position is always unique and beyond compare. Listen to your heart or listen to your mind either way life moves on and carries you with it.

Perhaps this sounds a little fatalistic, but I certainly don't mean to suggest that one should do nothing or that one should follow the suggested medical investigation route without complaint. One must follow the path with a heart and by that I mean that one must make the decision that seems most appropriate for your own particular philosophy and approach to life. There should be no judgement in this process or in the consequences of one's actions. Life is far too mysterious for anyone to know what is right or wrong in any particular situation.

Follow the path with a heart.

From the moment of birth we are moving like an arrow towards the death of our physical body. At the same time, if we so wish, we may be moving towards a greater spiritual enlightenment and enrichment. For some the latter may be more important than the aging and dying of the body. Health and disease are polarities like the two sides of a single coin. One cannot exist without the other.

Health attempts to prevent disease from becoming excessive and disease brings change into health, keeping it dynamic and creative. This is their relationship.

Chapter 13

One of my great delights as a schoolboy of 13 years old was to take small insects and place them under the microscope my father had bought me on my birthday. Looking down the lens was like entering another world. The insects became transformed into magical beasts with fascinating projections and mysterious moving parts. I was amazed that something so small had even smaller parts and I would carefully dissect these parts in order to discover what was inside.

The Human Anatomy Revisited

Can you see me? Can you Describe what a Human Being Looks Like?

Most of us believe that we know what human beings look like yet those descriptions are usually of the body. Are we bodies only and is sodium, potassium, cholesterol, fat, carbohydrate and protein etc. all that there is? Are we expected to believe that these physical substances are able to think and feel, have points of views and even believe in God?

If I am angry you can see on my face that I am angry, but it is not my face that is angry. So who is angry and where is that person? If my hand reaches out to touch you, it is not the muscles of the hand that have made this decision. So who is the operator?

Medical science has trapped us in its own limitations and instead of going on our own experience we had tended to disregard our own inner dialogue and opted instead to believe the limited viewpoint of science. What medical science can measure is chemistry and anatomy and because most research grants in medicine are directed by pharmaceutical companies who have a vested interest in chemistry the boundaries of our knowledge in human anatomy do not extend very far beyond what can be measured by biochemists and anatomists.

Most of us simple human beings live a strange paradox. We have almost begun to believe that human beings are nothing more that chemical factories which somehow are responsible for our emotions and that thought is a by-product of chemicals transported in the brain and nerve processes. Science may even one day be able to produce human beings in factories. Once the genetic code is broken then this reality it is believed is within our grasp.

On the other hand however a large majority of us believe in spirit and a God that is not physical and yet is able to influence physical events. A friend of mine is both a reborn Christian and a Professor of Engineering. So how does he deal with this paradox? The fact is that he keeps these two belief systems apart. When he thinks about God he must take his science hat off and when he deal with science then the rules of mathematics becomes his god. Einstein who was also a religious and spiritual man said that God does not play dice with the universe, meaning that intrinsic laws govern the universe, or is the universe itself dynamic, creative and intelligent? God does not play dice with the universe.

This was his dilemma with some of the new insights that were coming out of quantum mechanics that suggested a much more creative universe than the accepted Newtonian model recognised at the time. What Einstein meant was that in the physical world of matter and energy God had imprinted certain laws that were fixed and immutable so that the world ran like a clockwork and was governed by these laws which were imprinted on all living and non living things, in the way the planets moved around each other, the way the seasons flowed and weather changed. Certainly very complex, but nevertheless governed by law.

Some scientist even like to dwell on the possibility that in time they will be able to come up with a universal field theory that will encompass all the possible laws of the universe. This universal field theory would be the reflection of God's mind and perhaps was even God. God was a mathematical formula and once scientists understood that formula they could take over God's functions. Carl Sagan, the well know astronomer, is reputed to have said that with a universal field theory, who needs God?

The Clockwork Universe Running according to Fixed Immutable Laws

In the previous chapter we already alluded to the fact that human beings are not just a chemical soup but also electrical and magnetic fields and potentials. In this chapter I would like to look at what further evidence we have for these electrical currents and electromagnetic fields in order to enlarge our viewpoint of man as more than just a body as understood by conventional biology.

So, again we must continue our journey trying to link science and our experience with evidence that is close at hand. For this we must return to energy.

We know that there are electrical energies moving around the body and even magnetic fields. The Magnetoencephalogram is a measurement of the magnetic field within and around the brain and can even be measured at a distance away from the brain itself. The billions of heart cells beating in unison produce two and half watts of electrical energy with each heart beat; enough to light a small electric bulb.

One of the real pioneers of electromagnetism in biological systems is Dr Robert Becker, a Professor of Surgery, who has published a number of books on the subject. He was fascinated with the subject of regeneration in which certain animals such as the lizard and salamander are able to regrow body parts.

What he was able to demonstrate and confirm was that at an amputation site there was in fact a current of injury, which could be easily measured. It was always believed however that this current was a by-product of the chemistry of healing happening at the injured site. The current of injury was present in all animals, but what Dr Becker was able to show was that this current of injury had a negative potential in the salamander that was able to regenerate limbs and organs, but positive in the frog that could not.

He also demonstrated that this current of injury was measurable all the time the repair was taking place. These remarkable findings suggested that it was not just a simple matter of charged ions leaking across damaged membranes because the currents were different in the salamander and frog, but also the current continued all through the healing process and did not stop within a few days of the injury.

Dr Becker made the following astonishing statements:

'The electric currents I measured were active agents deliberately produced and directly related to the type of growth process the animal used to heal its wound. The control system that started, regulated, and stopped healing was electrical.'

This is an extraordinary statement made by a Professor of Medicine, that the electrical currents directed the healing process and one would imagine that scientists would be rushing out to try and prove or disprove his work. In fact very little money has been made available for such research and private individuals have done almost all such work.

Electrical currents direct and control the healing of wounds, said Dr Becker

The Chinese have practised acupuncture for thousands of years and despite efforts by scientists to discover the underlying chemical mechanism, there has not been much success. Most scientists are in agreement with the endorphin theory, which suggests that the needles stimulate the release of endorphins, which are morphine like chemicals, and this contributes to the pain relief seen in acupuncture.

This theory however does not make much sense to those who practise acupuncture. Patients receiving acupuncture usually come twice per week for treatment and as the condition improves the treatment is extended to once per week and then perhaps a few more treatments at longer intervals. With each treatment the pain becomes less intense and eventually disappears.

This is not the natural outcome when one uses drugs for symptomatic relief. Drugs must be taken at regular intervals and for prolonged periods of time. Symptom relief may be quick but healing is not the general outcome of drug use. If the drug is stopped the symptoms return.

Most people come to acupuncturists because their condition has not improved despite the usual medical treatment. Even morphine, a very powerful drug for pain, only works for some hours and does not heal anyone. Acupuncture stimulates healing and after each treatment there is an improvement, which is sustained for a longer and longer period until healing occurs. The ancient texts claim that the underlying problem in disease is the energetic disturbance and that by correcting this energetic disturbance a process of healing is induced and the symptoms improve.

The wind cannot be seen; only the movement of the leaves. One cannot find the wind by cutting open the leaf. If a person is angry one can see on their face that they are angry but the face is not angry. Nor can one find the person by dissecting the face. Electrical currents direct the healing of the amputated limb. Acupuncture is an energetic phenomenon and the healing is directed by changes in the flow of energy.

It has been demonstrated that acupuncture points can be measured with an ohmmeter and these points have been shown to have lowered skin resistance. They function as electrical windows into the system. The fact that the body may be penetrated through and through by electrical currents and electromagnetic fields should not come as a surprise.

There are billions of cells in the body with just as many complex biochemical processes and the whole must be co-ordinated in order to maintain the temperature, pH and other functions harmonised and balanced within very narrow limits. It is not possible for chemicals alone to move fast enough through the system to maintain this kind of order.

Dr. Valerie Hunt is a research scientist in neurophysiology and psychology with a special interest in the neuromuscular patterns of emotions. She spent many years studying the relationship between emotions and the electric conduction in muscles. Wires needed to be attached to the person which were cumbersome and perhaps disturbed the results.

She later used a system developed by NASA called Telemetry, which used a radio broadcasting system capable of intercepting and projecting the body's electric activity. She reported that Telemetry allowed a small, continuous millivolt signal to be recorded from the body surface unlike any she had seen before. Of special interest was that this field responded before the brain wave activity was noted and before stimuli altered the heart rate, blood pressure or breathing.

It was as if '......the primary response in this world takes place first in the auric field, neither in the sensory nerves nor in the brain.' She called this field of activity the auric field as she had already been working with a number of 'sensitives' who could 'see' such fields.

Telemetry Signals Preceded all other Recordings from the Body

What may be astonishing to many readers is the fact that vast numbers of children and adults are able to see these energy fields around the body. These have been well described over thousands of years. The halo depicted around saints is an example of this. I have interviewed a number of very sane and common folk who can see these auras. My impression is that this gift is becoming more and more apparent and was certainly present in many individuals all around the world thousands of years ago.

Auras or Energy Fields can be Seen by Many Children and Adults

Dr Valerie Hunt reported that studies over 20 years established the reliability of these sensitives. She was able to make this claim after comparing simultaneous readings from eight experienced auric readers. Using her instruments she was also able to identify the wave patterns of a number of these energy fields and correlate them with the colours described by the sensitives.

'Throughout the centuries in which sensitives have seen and described the auric emissions, this is the first objective electronic evidence of frequency, amplitude and time, which validates their subjective observation of colour discharge.'

Dr. Barbara Ann Brennan is another physicist who has studied the aura. She is able to see the various auric fields which show up as different colours. Her physics background has given her a language with which to communicate this information to colleagues and other scientists.

'Our old world of solid concrete objects is surrounded by and permeated with a fluid world of radiating energy, constantly moving, constantly changing like the sea.'

Another person whose work should be mentioned is Professor Bjorn Nordenstrom, well known for his work on X-rays. He did extensive work on the body's electric current, which he claimed had a major influence on water transport, cell movement and other biological activities. He was even able to document regression of lung cancers using electrical currents directed through the cancer.

One may well ask why it is that this work is being sidelined if indeed there is anything in it. The sad truth is that all medical and biological research is to a large extend dependent on pharmaceutical companies which have no interest in research which is not maintaining and supporting the biochemical view of man.

As important to the role of major pharmaceutical companies is the role that universities have in controlling the depth of education in biology and medicine in particular. This is done through limiting curricular, regulatory and review committees that define the edges of what is allowed to be known and accepted and limiting investigation of what is regarded as forbidden territory.

What is allowed to be known and investigated by medical scientists is strictly limited.

Science draws its own boundaries to new discoveries.

Work is continuing mainly by private organizations and individuals .It however will require a critical mass of information to emerge before this kind of work becomes common knowledge. The following conclusions are based on my reading of the information and encounters of a personal kind:

- Human energy fields do exist and some can be measured.

- These energy fields interact with physiology and anatomy.

- The energy fields are open and respond creatively or sometimes destructively with biological tissue.

- The energy fields appear to connect to more subtle energy fields.

- These subtle energy fields may be what are referred to as mind, spirit and even consciousness.

- Changes in these energy fields seem to precede changes in physiology.

- Intent on the part of the healer can change the energy field of the patient and initiate a healing process.

More recent research confirms the fact that the human being and all living systems are functioning and influenced by fields beyond matter. Mae Wan Ho is a Ph.D in Biology and studies the coherent fields in living systems. He says the following:

'In the breath-taking colour images we generated, one can see that the activities of the organism are fully coordinated in a continuum from the macroscopic to the molecular. The organism is coherent beyond our wildest dreams. Every part is in communication with every other part through a dynamic, tuneable, responsive, liquid crystalline medium that pervades the whole body, from organs and tissues to the interior of every cell. Liquid crystallinity gives organisms their characteristic flexibility, exquisite sensitivity and responsiveness, this optimising

the rapid intercommunication that enables the organism to function as a coherent whole.'[1]

Intent on the part of the healer can change the energy field of the patient and initiate a healing process

This latter statement does require some further explanation and will be discussed in other chapters. It is an extremely important observation and perhaps account for the fact that some practitioners get much better results than colleagues using the same techniques.

The work of the HeartMath organisation has shown that negative emotions lead to increased disorder in the heart's rhythms and in the autonomic nervous system, thereby adversely affecting the rest of the body. In contrast, positive emotions create increased harmony and coherence in heart rhythms and improve balance in the nervous system.

Dr. Popp in Germany has spent years demonstrating that living systems emit and absorb photons. Using a sensitive photon detector this is not difficult to measure. He believes that light within the body might even hold a key to health and ill health. It has a great deal to do with resonance, frequency, amplitude and fields of activity. This is so exceedingly complex that most researchers don't want to spend time doing the work required.

Again the work by brave scientists is dismissed. A massive pharmacological industry is at stake, a worldview of how the body works is being challenged and so for now we are left with biochemistry running the show.

The ECG (electromagnetic recording of the heart) and EEG (electromagnetic recording of the brain) are merely dismissed as interesting electrical recordings, which primarily are by-products of biochemistry and otherwise have no physiological repercussions on the body and are secondary phenomena (i.e. appear after the physiological recordings).

1   Mae Wan Ho " The Entangled Universe", Yes! A
     Journal of Positive Futures, Spring 2000

So this very complex heart electrical process which runs through the whole body right down to the toes and up into the head and can even be measured some distance outside the body is just that- a recording telling doctors about the status of the heart. It seems strange indeed that scientists assume that this complex reading merely passes through every cell and tissue of the body without having any effect, does not carry information to each cell and is not the way the heart also collects information back from the body.

What about memory and how is memory stored. Again we have no problem is recognising that information can be stored as information in our computers, downloaded and transferred without any chemicals involved. So why do scientists struggle to understand memory in living systems.

The problem again is about going beyond the limited chemical profiling of living systems and recognising the energy-informational system that needs to be appended to the biochemistry. In other words the human being, as are all living systems, is a matter-energy-informational system.

Right now the controversy looks something like this:

Human beings are primary matter (physical and biochemical) with some energy and information aspects resulting from matter.

Or

Human beings are primarily energy-informational systems, which control matter.

The side you take will give some clue to the way you think about the world.

I believe that we have energy and information, which has an enormous influence on the body, and that what happens in the body has a resonance into the energy-information. These ideas allow me to have clearer understanding about the mind (energy-information) and the brain (matter) and to understand how the ego or personality can slowly gather information around itself to create the sense of 'I' and how this 'I' can influence the matter/body.

We can now make the following statements regarding the anatomy of human beings. Men and woman are not bodies which have learnt to feel and think. Instead they are energy-informational beings that have a physical body to work with.

Some of these energies can be easily measured although we have not yet learnt to understand exactly what their function is and how they interact with other fields. It is important to keep in mind that scientists know very little about magnetic and electrical fields anyway.

We know how to use these fields but very little else is known about them. They remain an enigma. The human energy fields are not any different. They are there but medical science has not yet even acknowledged their existence as anything more than a by-product of physiology. Since ancient times however they have been well described and have been given various names.

Paracelsus, a renaissance philosopher and healer has written that...'there exists another half of man: man does not consist of flesh and blood alone, but also of a body that cannot be discerned by our crude eyesight'. Humans have bodies both visible and invisible. The happiness can be seen on the face but it is not the face that is happy.

Dissecting the muscles of the face or sending blood or other material from the face to the laboratory will not help either to identify the source of the happiness or the person that is happy. We are mysterious beings and we need to claim back our mystery as part of who we are even though science cannot resolve this enigma of 'life' and the vast territory beyond 'matter' itself.

Science has disempowered us by suggesting that human beings are only that which science can and wants to measure, which is biochemistry and anatomy. The research of the ancients and the experience of many human beings today attest to a much more complex and grand design.

Ken Wilber in his book 'The marriage of sense and soul' speaks of reality being 'a rich tapestry of interwoven levels... reaching from matter to body to soul to spirit. Each senior level 'envelops' or 'enfolds' its junior dimensions. A series of nests within nests within nests within nests of being. So that everything and events in the world is interwoven with every other.'

The human being can be understood best in the same way. It is in fact our experience of ourselves. A physical/chemical body permeated and surrounded by an energetic body, an emotional energetic body of colour (red with anger, green with jealousy), a mind body of two interlinking functional parts often referred to as the 'left brain' logical thinking part and 'right brain' intuitive part.

All this suffused by and surrounded by the subtlest body of each person's spirit and soul. Finally connected to the infinite body of God/Tao/quantum potential/Consciousness or whatever other name you want to call 'Infinity'. The 'Body' of God and the body of human beings are at last connected clearly through finer and finer energy bodies.

Anatomy - Biochemistry - Electromagnetism - Subtle Bodies (mind, spirit, soul) - Consciousness.

I am playing around with words here and trying to make the point that we need to be careful not to get too stuck on our particular definition of words so that we don't see the connections and similarity of what we are referring to. There is so much commonality between what many people call 'God' and others call 'consciousness' or the 'Tao' that it seems unwise to be too dogmatic around these definitions and seek rather the common themes that unite.

One more point needs to be clarified i.e. the difference between mind and brain. Without the energetic understanding these two words are often confused or used to mean the same thing. Brain is very obviously the physical substance within the skull but does the word include the magnetic field measured around the brain; and how do we understand consciousness and where is the thinker.

Clarity is restored when we understand that these latter words refer not to the brain itself but to the mind, which is one of the subtle energy fields. Thus to refer to the left and right brain is somewhat confusing. There is not enough substantial difference in the left and right brain to account for the kind of difference in function that is usually given to these areas. Instead left and right brain really refers to the two primary functions of mind i.e. the logical rational mind and the intuitive creative artistic mind.

So sit down quietly in a chair, feel your body relax, take in a few deep breaths and with each outbreath feel yourself relaxing more and more. Bring up this question 'Who am I?' Feel your body on the chair and your breathing in and out and notice that there is someone having the experience of body. So who is this person who seems not to be the body?

Notice your thoughts, as they clearly appear to move like streams of energy in the head area and emotions, which also move like streams of energy in the body. It is an assumption and not science to believe that somehow all the known functions of human beings are all initiated by biochemistry.

Depression, anxiety and other emotional states cannot be diagnosed by taking a blood specimen and sending it to the laboratory. Biochemistry does not have the complexity to describe human behaviour and creativity. While biochemistry is itself complex there is nothing within its physical properties which suggests that it can think and feel and have emotions.

Suggesting an energetic template behind the biochemical processes not only makes sense but is supported by the experience of many individuals as described above and can be measured today with sensitive instruments. This would go a long way to bridging the gap between our understanding of a human being as anatomy and biochemistry and spirit.

There are other areas of experience, even common every day experience, which points to our energy fields extending away from the body. Notice for example how uncomfortable or comfortable you feel standing closer or further from certain people.

The electromagnetic field of the heart radiates out almost a metre beyond our body itself. What does that say about heart to heart conversations? Notice how certain areas, different trees; places in your garden all affect you differently.

All is energy and we are all energetic beings. When the truth of this understanding again becomes known as it has been known throughout the ages then humankind will make giant steps in all direction, not least in medicine and the ability to understand health and disease.

Matter and Energy Make Way for Information

Having bridged the gap from body-material substance across to energy we are now ready to make one further move in trying to understand intelligence and consciousness.

Just as an electrical wire to a TV set has no special interest if all it does is give us the means to switch the set on and off, so the physical brain and energy fields would have no special interest if consciousness was not present. What makes the TV set so exciting is the information carried by the electrical current and appearing on the screen. Similarly

173

the mind is not only an energy field but also moves information around. It is the presence of this information that makes consciousness, thinking, self- awareness and intuition possible.

So our anatomy of human beings begins to look like this:

- Body (anatomy + physiology)

- Energy (electromagnetic + non-measurable subtle energy such as emotions)

- Information (consciousness, thought, intuition)

While the brain is confined to the head region Mind is not localized here and for this reason left and right brain is a convention only but a misleading one at that.

Mind has probably both energetic and information components.

Perhaps we can go into the experience of this so I ask readers again to sit down, close the eyes and become silent for a few minutes breathing deeply in and out.

Now try and get a sense of where thinking happens. Where would you point to when saying 'I think that'...

Now where would you place your hand when saying 'I feel deep in my heart that...?'

Now how about this one

'My gut feeling is that...'

Or

'Wow, isn't that an attractive man...? '

Our experience is clearly that mind is not localized to the brain area only. Thinking takes place in the head area but feeling and a deep knowingness seems to be closer to the chest/heart area while our gut or instinctive area is below the diaphragm as is our sexual experience.

Head = Thinking

Throat = Expression

Heart = Feeling

Head/Heart = Intuition

Abdomen = Instinct / Gut Feeling

Groin = Sex

Below the diaphragm is our more animal instinctual nature related to fear and flight, hunting and seeking and procreation. Above the diaphragm the mind functions have to do with feeling and thinking.

It is important that we allow our experience to become part of what we know and work with and not rely only on scientists to inform us about the nature of reality. The world is so complex and linked together is many subtle ways that conventional science can only give evidence of a very small part of the whole

Conclusions

- Biochemistry is not enough information to understand health and ill health. It is only one very narrow entry into the whole human being and his or her experience.

- Electromagnetic energy is everywhere and absolutely necessary to run computers, motor cars, machinery of all types, alarm systems, opening and closing gates, electricity etc. It is also everywhere in the human body.

- We live in an information age and respect the powerful place for information as the controlling, directing and transferring bits that make sense of the electromagnetic fields.

- Matter-energy-information (MEI) is the greater 'anatomy' of the human being and as we allow the enormous work which has already been performed in this field to be incorporated into medicine and shift away from the focus on 'chemical' medicine we will find it much easier to shift ill health using the astonishingly sophisticated research of physicists and engineers everywhere.

Chapter 14

The Healing Process

What does the Healing Process need to Function Well?

A s indicated repeatedly in this book, 'healing' is an innate self-motivating and intelligent homeostatic mechanism in the body.

Healing is a Self-motivating, Intelligent and Homeostatic Natural Process

Any system of healing is finally dependent on what the systems in the body can do to heal. Keep reminding yourself also that when I refer to the 'body' I always mean the body in the greater anatomy sense of:

Body-emotions-mind-spirit-consciousness and Matter-energy-information-quantum space

This is the human being as a whole functioning system. The 'disease' or ill health will always involved the whole system. When you stub your toe, the whole body knows about it and while the swelling may be localised, nevertheless this is a response from the system as a whole. Nothing will happen in an isolated way.

Antibiotics don't heal the system but kill bacteria. The body still must do the healing. Nutrients don't heal the system but provide the system with the nutrients it needs to heal itself. The surgeon does not heal anyone but merely assists by removing an obstruction, a cancer or corrects a problem and makes it sometimes easier for the body to heal. At the end of the day everyone is exhausted and eventually goes to sleep.

During the night the body's systems are able to function without the interference of mental-emotional stuff or more food requiring digestion so that the greater anatomy indicated above does its best to return the system back to good functionality. We wake up refreshed and ready for the day after going to bed exhausted and non functional.

The ancients understood the basics i.e. that a good nights sleep and rest was important when a person was ill. Drink lots of water to keep the systems ability to remove toxins flowing and remove the person from stress. Herbs were used to support the healing and there was also the intrinsic understanding that for some people just touching them kindly, gently rubbing the body with oils had beneficial qualities and improved healing.

Today with the knowledge we have of physiology and biochemistry there is a greater understanding what is required to improve and optimize function. Holistic doctors take these processes into account when deciding on how to manage the ill health and disease. Rather than focusing on the 'disease', these practitioners decide on what functions are no longer operating optimally and initiate processes to help the innate healing processes return the system to normal healthy functions.

Let's have a look at some of the mechanisms required for optimum healing.

a: An intact and functioning immune system.

The immune system is our great defence system spread throughout the body with a special concentration in the area of the gastro-intestinal tract. This is not surprising. The lumen of the GIT contains contaminated contents from outside the body, which are constantly in the process of breaking down and being absorbed, and passing to the liver for filtering. Between the GIT and the liver sits 60% of the immune cells in what is referred to as peyers patches.

Collectively these are also called the gut-associated lymphoid tissue (GALT) and consist of isolated or aggregated immune system cells. These are the immune sensors of the intestine and are constantly monitoring both antigenic material and pathogenic micro-organism coming from the intestines.

This makes complete sense if we understand the importance of preventing micro-organism present in massive amounts in the GIT from entering into the cellular spaces of the body. In addition the food must be broken down into its smallest components so that it no longer carries the identity of the original living substance from which it is derived.

How amazing is that! We all know that doctors cannot transplant an organ, blood or other tissues from another person unless they are compatible because of the ability of the body to reject foreign material.

In a similar way the body's digestive processes make sure that what is passing down the GIT has all its 'personal labels' removed right down to its basic structures so that there is nothing recognizable from its original source. That is quite an accomplishment and a marvellous piece of engineering.

If for some reason gaps begin to appear between the cells of the intestinal tract known as 'leaky gut' then food particles which have not been adequately digested can pass through causing immune system over-reaction leading to food allergic reactions and even autoimmune disease in which the body become self destructive.

Many diseases are thought to arise in this way such as Systemic lupus erythematosis (SLE), Rheumatoid arthritis, multiple sclerosis, type 1 diabetes and many other conditions.

What are the requirements for the immune system to function optimally? A study of biochemistry or physiology will alert the reader to the vitamins, minerals, amino acids, essential fatty acids and other nutrients required to optimise a healthy response. These are not drug deficiency problems but an inadequate supply of nutrients or other factors interfering with normal function.

What is required for healthy immune function is the basic building blocks for the chemicals, which are used to constitute the enzymes, hormones, prostaglandins, proteins and all the other chemical compounds required for normal function. If there is a deficiency of any one of these basic chemicals then the immune system will be stressed and not function optimally. These basic nutrient requirements are derived from the food, water and air that are taken into the body.

The level of health of the immune system will to a large extent decide who will fall ill during an epidemic, how long it takes for full blown AIDS to develop and how fast it progresses. The health of the immune system will also decide on our recovery after an operation, how long it takes and whether serious complications develop.

Even our response to vaccinations is dependent on a healthy immune system and this is why the influenza vaccine does not work very well in babies and old people whose immune systems are either not yet well developed or becoming more inefficient.

Like all other systems in the body, nutrients are essential for immune function. Nutrients become the enzymes, immune factors, cell walls, nerves, brain and heart etc. It is why we eat, drink and breathe.

178

The immune system has a particular need for certain nutrients. Patrick Bouic, professor of immunology at Stellenbosch medical school, Cape Town, South Africa, discusses ten nutritional supplements that are essential in his book 'The Immune system cure'. They include vitamin A, B6, C, E, magnesium, selenium, zinc, coenzyme Q10, Reduced L-glutathione and DHEA.

For those unwilling or unable to eat lots of fresh organic fruit and vegetables then supplementation is essential.

Junk food and fast foods are nutritionally deficient and clearly do not optimize the immune system. They must be eliminated from the diet if one wants to have a well functioning immunity. Taking drugs is not the answer to immune deficiency. Antibiotics can assist in a serious infection but if the immune system is in poor health then a resolution of the infection may be inadequate, long and protracted.

The strength and resilience of the immune system varies enormously from birth to old age and is influenced by many factors. The baby's immunity and general health is dependent on the mother's health and diet, and the immune system develops its resilience from contact with the environment and micro-organisms it comes in contact with.

Parents often ask me about the best way to stimulate and strengthen the immune system. Apart from good food and appropriate supplements, childhood infectious diseases are probably the natural way the immune system was challenged and developed good resistance for later in life. Excessive use of antibiotics is generally unnecessary, not supportive and interferes with the natural process of developing this necessary resistance.

All infectious disease including the common influenza is powerful stimulants of the immune system and these infections may even strengthen the body against cancer in later life.

With aging there is a serious decrease in a number of critical immune system components including cellular response, antibody production and response to vaccines. For this reason, as already stated, vaccinations don't seem to work well in older individuals.

Older people suffer from chronic disease, chronic inflammation and cancer suggesting an immune dysfunction at work underlying many of the diseases doctors see in their practice.

Malnutrition and psychological health also affects the immune system.

Stress and anxiety can increase the production of pro-inflammatory chemicals, which means that the immune system is inappropriately on high alert. Chronic overproduction of inflammatory chemicals can do damage to the normal structures of the body.

The immune system can be over-stimulated or even suppressed. An example of chronic stress suppressing the immune system is that of caregivers looking after a relative with serious medical conditions, which can result in long-term immune suppression among the caregivers. The same applies to persistent marital problems, burnout at work and lengthy unemployment.

Parents sometimes get overinvolved in cleanliness, believing that they must protect their children from germs. Yet studies have shown that children brought up on family-scale farms, drinking raw milk and living close to farm animals generally tend to have less allergies, asthma and other autoimmune problems compared to children raised away from farm environments.

Children who never spent any time on a farm in one study were nearly three times as likely as farm-raised children to develop allergies. As one of the researchers involved in this study said 'People have grown up with animals and in outdoor environments for eons, and maybe our immune systems are tuned to developing normally in that sort of environment'.

I have seen parents, especially those living in the city, overinvolved in keeping their children away from 'unclean' things, washing their children's hands continuously after touching door handles etc., but they don't seem to realise that much more important than this is keeping the child's nutritional levels optimised to the best of their ability.

The elderly should also be concerned about their immune system's health, which tends to become inefficient with age. Simple infections can very quickly become life threatening and cancer and other chronic diseases are also much more common.

The elderly living in old age homes in particular often have very poor diets and suffer from major nutrient deficiencies. Imagine how much the chronic disease burden could be reduced by supplementing the elderly with a good quality nutritional mix, which supports immune health.

Acute infections can be life threatening in any age but it is exactly these acute responses that activate the immune system and set the tone for future immune reactions and health of the system as a whole.

Natural approaches to support the immune response can work as powerfully, as fast and generally more effectively than drugs. The latter should be used only when natural methods no longer are working or the system's response is inadequate to deal with the attack from outside or inside or if the condition is life threatening and a powerful response is required. Nevertheless one always needs to consider the risk vs the benefits of drug us.

Chronic inflammation is a different condition. Not only are pro-inflammatory chemicals constantly being produced, but also there is an increased concentration of free radicals with their unpaired electrons looking for available electrons.

Free radicals can cause serious damage by reacting with other molecules, changing their chemical composition, damaging fat, proteins and nucleic acids. They can cause cell death, gene mutations and cancer. Chronic inflammation is linked to heart disease, brain damage and many other problems.

Important to keep the following in mind:

• Food choices: Fresh organic food is packed with immune supporting nutrients, which are generally removed, decreased or chemically distorted by processing.

• Sugar suppresses the immune system.[1] 100gm portions of carbohydrate from glucose, fructose, sucrose, honey or orange juice significantly decreased the capacity of neutrophils to engulf bacteria for 1-2 hours postprandial, but were still present to some degree at 5 hours.

• Exercise has a positive influence on the immune system; nevertheless it is important to recognise that serious exercise for prolonged periods can generates a great deal of free radicals. On

1   Sanchez A et al Role of sugars in human neutrophil phagocytosis.Am J Clin Nutr 1973; 26:1180-1184

the days I go to the gym I add extra anti-oxidants to my usual supply.

- A good night's sleep is important for immune system health.

- Laughter, relaxation all helps immune health.

Other important nutrients

- Vitamin D: Children and adults with higher vitamin D levels contract fewer colds and other viral infections. Vitamin D down-regulates the expression of pro- inflammatory cytokines and up-regulates the expression of antimicrobial peptides in immune cells.

- Glutamine is the most abundant amino acid in the body. It has immune-regulative properties and lymphocytes and macrophages use glutamine at a very high rate. Endurance athletes who do not fully recover between workouts have decreased glutamine levels.

- SAMe (S-adenosyl-L-methionine): Natural amino acid present in the body and linked to the synthesis of glutathione, the body's most important anti-oxidant.

- NAC (N-Acetyl-Cysteine): also linked to the production of glutathione. 600-1800mg/day

- Lipoic acid: important anti-oxidant because soluble in fat and water. Anti-viral, free radical quenching and immune boosting qualities.

- Whey protein: has precursor amino acids for the synthesis of glutathione. Also contains key substances to enhance immune system, which include: beta-lactoglobulin, alpha-lactalbumin, lactoperoxidase, and lactoferrin. Whey protein can activate natural killer cells.

- Bovine Colostrum: This is the first milk produced by cows during the first several days post parturition. It contains high amounts of immunoglobulin, growth factors, and immune cytokines. It is also rich in antimicrobial and immune regulating factors. One of its functions is to seriously activate the baby's immune system coming into contact with the outside world for the first time.

- Omega 3. An imbalance between the ratio of omega 3:6 has been associated with increasing inflammation. Counteracts suppression of cellular immunity.

- Probiotics. The connection with the bacterial flora in the gastro-intestinal tract and immune system (GALT) is interesting and suggests a kind of interactive connection, keeping the immune system dynamic and robust. Each day we produce several ounces of bacteria and eliminate several ounces in the bowel action. There is an enormous turnover and yet a remarkable stability at the same time. Dietary choices may promote co-operation between humans and the gut microbes or even promote conflict leading to inflammation and other metabolic disturbances. Western type diets with low fibre content, high in simple sugars, saturated fats and emulsifying agents may contribute to human disease because they do not support the health of the microbiome.

Studies indicate that children born to families who consume traditional Lactobacillus-rich fermented foods experience fewer allergies than those from families who consume more sterile foods.

- Grape seed extract (proanthocyanidins) have antioxidant and immune-boosting properties. 150mg/day

- Green tea extract: antioxidant and free radical-scavenging abilities. Also has anticancer effects, modulates inflammation and protects against DNA damage.

- Andrographis: a herb used in Asia and India to treat infections, inflammations, colds and fevers. Its effects seem to be at the bone marrow and spleen levels.

- Garlic 1200mg/d

- Thymus extract

Does the mind have any influence on the immune system?

In the chapter on the placebo response I have documented many clinical studies showing the effect of a placebo and healing responses. The placebo is so effective that all drug trials require the placebo as a control. Hypnosis is another area showing the powerful effects of the mind over the body.

Research has also shown that meditation is an effective method for a variety of physical and mental disorders including chronic pain, cardiovascular disease, skin disorders and other conditions.

None of this should be surprising. It doesn't need research to know and experience the effects of mind over body. A simple thought raises the hand; the stress of going to a doctor to have the blood pressure taken can increase the blood pressure substantially. Any emotion can be felt in the body and causes disruption of function. These disruptions of function can manifest as spastic colon, irritable bowel, headaches, tiredness, loss of appetite, shoulder/neck stiffness and pain etc.

The immune system does age over time. What this means is that its ability to respond effectively to stress diminishes.

Summary

- Immune system does not need antibiotics.

- Sugar also weakens immune response

- Food choices do make a difference

- Nutrients are essential for immune response: omega 3 (anti-inflammatory), zinc, selenium, vitamin A, vitamin D, colostrum.

- Sleep and exercise support immune function

b: The organs of elimination are functioning effectively

The organs of elimination include the liver, kidney, lungs, skin and mucous membrane. Even without all the environmental toxins taken into the body there are bye products of metabolic processes happening in the body which are poisonous and must be eliminated. This is a continuous process of detoxification and is essential to good health. This requires some elaboration.

The liver is the chief detoxification organ acting as an important filter of the blood. Detoxification has two phases, One and Two. During phase One, fat-soluble toxins must be made water soluble for elimination but in that process more toxins are generated. If these toxins are not rapidly removed by phase 2 then they can accumulate and pass back into the blood stream. This process of moving toxins through the liver can be interfered with or become inefficient in people with fatty livers, drinking excess alcohol, which is a liver poison, and poor nutritional status required for optimum liver function.

The two phases of the liver require a range of nutrients to function normally as can be seen in the diagram below.

Toxins → Phase 1 →	Phase 2 →	Waste Products
(fat soluble)		(water soluble)
Phase 1 Required Nutrients	**Phase 2 Required Nutrients**	↓
Folic Acid	Calcium d-Glucarate	Eliminated from the body via:
Vitamin B3	Amino acids:	↓ ↓
Vitamin B6	L-glutamine	Gall bladder ↓
Vitamin B12	L-lysine HCL	↓ Kidneys
Vitamin A	Glycine	Bile ↓
Vitamin C	L-carnitine	↓ Urine ↓
Calcium	Taurine	Bowel Action
Vitamin D3	Cruciferous vegetable (sulphur metabolites)	
Vitamin E	MSM	
Milk Thistle	N-acetyl Cysteine	
N-acetyl Cysteine		
Citrus bioflavinoids		
Quercetin		
Toxin list		
Metabolic end products	Contaminants/ polutants	
Micro-organisms	Food additives	
Pesticides	Drugs	
Insecticides	Alcohol	

What is required for the detoxification process is a good supply of nutrients, not drugs. A deficiency of any one nutrient can decrease the efficiency of the process and means increasing toxins that must be handled by the body and possibly stored in the fatty tissues. Even a casual look at the list will make it obvious why Integrative doctors pay so much attention to this process. Almost all the vitamins required are seriously deficient in our diets.

Is it possible that one of the reasons for increasing obesity is the need by the body to find a depository for all these fat-soluble toxins that must be removed from the circulation? This may also account for the fact that some people have such difficulty in loosing weight.

Fat tissue is a storehouse of toxins.

It is not only in the liver that chemicals, which could be toxic, are produced but all over the body there are metabolic processes that include a phase that produce chemicals which could cause problems. An example is the methylation process.

Methylation has a range of processes essential to health including the production of glutathione which is perhaps one of the most important anti-oxidants. The cycle from methionine to glutathione produces homocysteine, which many doctors believe may be a more important chemical than cholesterol, causing atherosclerosis and heart disease. The methylation cycle to function efficiently requires folic acid, B12, B6 and some amino acids.

Again we see the key role of nutrients for metabolic functionality. Without these nutrients, homocysteine could accumulate and the person could end up with heart disease. Treating the heart disease and ignoring the methylation problem is clearly not a holistic answer to management. It is what I call treating the 'end point' diagnosis rather than the underlying dysfunction.

Many of these chemicals of breakdown are toxic and must be removed fairly rapidly. So here we have it. The internal production of toxic chemicals on the way to being removed, and if not eliminated can cause symptoms and serious disturbances even death. Such an extreme example would be someone in diabetic coma. The cause is chemicals generated in the body that cannot be removed rapidly enough. Less obvious causes are over-eating causing serious body discomforts due to the accumulating toxins generated by the digestion, absorption and breakdown of food.

The intelligence of this system is surprising. Despite the hundreds if not thousands of new chemicals added into the environment every year the organs of elimination do a very good job at findings ways to remove them away from vital organs and functions provided that the system is working well.

The diagram above gives a pretty good idea of what is required to improve liver detoxification . There are many other ways to assist detoxification in the body. These include sweating(exercise, Sauna etc), Epsom salt baths, massage which helps to drain the lymphatic system, juice fasting, eating vegetable and fruit only, adding fibre to the diet.

c: A Normal Healthy Flora within the Intestinal Tract

Today it is no longer enough to just refer to the flora in the intestinal tract. There is also micro-organism on the skin, micro-organisms covering all other mucous membranes such as the sinuses, nasal cavity, and vagina. A new term 'the microbiome' has emerged to include all these micro-organisms in addition to viruses and fungi. There are more living organisms in the microbiome than all the cells of the body and this also constitutes a higher proportion of DNA particles that that of the body itself.

Imagine this microbiome is like a flock of birds flying through the sky. They have a kind of cohesion, connecting to each other moving in a most harmonious way.

There are more bacteria in our intestinal tract than cells in our body with 400 to 500 types and many different strains. Twenty types make up three-quarters of the total. These include the well-known lactobacillus and bifidobacteria but also bacteroides, eubacterium, fusobacteria, peptococcacaceae and streptococcus.

Some are aerobic (need oxygen) and some anaerobic (don't need oxygen) and there are also lactic acid-producing bacteria. The latter, by producing lactic acid, keep the contents of the colon slightly acidic and protect us from the overgrowth of harmful bacteria. The weight of this intestinal flora is about 1,5kg, which is about equal to the weight of the liver.

There is a constant turnover of bacteria as many are discarded with each bowel action. This is a most complex and intricate collection of not just bacteria but also viruses, fungi and even parasites living together in a fine balance that is maintained throughout the person's life.

It seems that the body actually nourishes the microbes to maintain their health and perhaps even consolidate the growth of certain species. As one researcher says:[2]

'Our gut microbes are not just passive recipients of the food that we eat – they evolve and change in response to what we feed our bodies. There are certain foods that lead to resource sharing between us and our microbes, while other foods can lead to conflict and resource competition between our bodies and our microbes,' Aktipis says. 'This co-operation and conflict framework can help us understand certain aspects of why we get sick and how we can stay healthy.'

We are born with a sterile internal environment but even as we pass through the mother's vagina the baby is confronted with and is invaded by a range of the mother's micro- organisms. Our external environment is certainly not sterile and very quickly invades the baby's skin and enters other orifices. This is all a natural process that has evolved over time.

The food choices we make will also affect the types of bacteria flora in the gastrointestinal tract and in turn also affect the health of the organism.

Lactobacilli are a very important group and found mainly in the small intestine while the bifidobacterium are found mainly in the colon.

The flora are essential to our health, just as bees are essential for pollination. They are a frontline in our immune defense by preventing colonization by pathogens and also manufacturing many vitamins for us, including some vitamin Bs, vitamin A and K.

Probiotics are supported by prebiotics. The latter bolster and promote the growth of the probiotics entering into the gastro-intestinal tract. They include products such as rice fibre, inulin and fructo-oligosaccherides (FOS) and arabinogalactans and include Jerusalem artichokes, onions, chicory, garlic, leeks, bananas, soybeans, asparagus, whole rye and whole-wheat.

2   Science Daily June 6, 2016

Beneficial Metabolic Effects of Enteric Microbiota:

- Biotransformation of bile acids.

- Production of micronutrients (eg vitamin K, biotin, folate)

- Participation in fermentation of otherwise indigestible polysaccharides by colonic bacteria to short chain fatty acids which are a major energy source for the colonic mucous membrane cells.

- Aiding in the metabolism and/or activation of medications

- Prevention of colonization in the gut by pathogenic microorganism.

- Bacterial enzymes play an important role in altering substances for chemical processes, e.g. blood level of estrogen is affected by bacterial enzyme.

Gut flora can promote health or even cause ill health.

- 90% of carcinogenic substances the human body is exposed to require chemical changes or bio activation before acting as a carcinogen. Imbalance in gut flora may play a key role in the development of certain cancers. (Bacteria can activate carcinogens)

- Antigenic substances produced by intestinal bacteria also appear related to the development of immune-related diseases. Inflammatory joint disease for example may be associated with immune complexes in the blood which arise from bacteria present in the gut lumen.

Keep in mind the following important relationships:

- The probiotic profile inherited from the mother via the delivery method.

- The disturbing effect of antibiotics on the microbiome. Note also that farmers use antibiotics in animals not only to deal with infections but also to fatten the animals. This may have the same effect on humans i.e excessive and prolong use of antibiotics may contribute to the obesity epidemic.

- The importance of fiber for gut health. The roles of dietary fiber, which promotes health by fueling beneficial bacteria to produce compounds that help, regulate the immune function. Processed and junk foods contain very little fibre. In the processing of refining wheat to make white flour the germ and bran are removed which contains most of the good health ingredients. That's not all of course. The grains are stored for long periods and require fungicides to prevent fungus growing and the flour is also bleached with chlorine gas to make it whiter and preserve it longer. Not exactly a health food.

Soluble fibre increases production of the anti-inflammatory protein interleukin-4 and shifts the immune system to anti-inflammatory mode. This could protect obese individuals from the inflammatory components of fat tissue.

Few people get the standard recommendation of 30 to 32 grams of fibre per day, and when fibre is lacking, it starves these beneficial bacteria, thereby setting your health into a downward spiral.

Soluble fibre is also converted to short-chain fatty acids (butyric acids), which in turn converted to healthy ketones that feed the tissues. These fibres essential to the health of gut bacteria, which in turn are essential to health of organism.

Insoluble fibre gives bulk to the contents of the bowel and can prevent constipation.

Soluble Fibre is food for the gut microbiome and is essential for health of the whole organism.

d: Optimum Nutritional Status

Nutrient deficiencies are a major problem on every continent and within all racial and population groups. The idea that somehow most of us are getting 'sufficient' nutrients in our diet is just not true.

Nutritional deficiencies are present throughout the population for many different reasons:

- Poor diet especially using refined foods deficient in nutrients. This is probably the most common reason for serious deficiencies. Junk food and refined food even when supplemented is inadequate nourishment. While some foods are supplemented with nutrients such as folic acid, the latter is synthetic and different to the more natural folate. As I keep pointing out similar is not exact and the body knows the difference.

• Imbalanced diet e.g. excess omega 6. This is due to all the processed oils used by everyone. Omega 6 oils are inflammatory promoting. Excess sugar is another cause of an imbalanced diet.

• Enzyme deficiencies preventing the use of nutrients. This deficiency may be genetic but also due to toxins and drugs interfering with enzyme function.

• Increased need for nutrients, e.g. fever, exercise or stress. The adrenals for example need lots of vitamin C when there is stress. Following surgery the body requires increasing amounts of vitamin C to heal the local wound.

Initially the stores of the various nutrients are used up, placing stress on the system, but no symptoms of ill health may yet occur. As the deficiency becomes worse physiological impairment arises leading in time to symptoms and signs.

While gross deficiencies are obvious, it is the much earlier phases of deficiencies that are difficult to identify especially when this involves more than one nutrient and the symptoms may only be tiredness, irritability, insomnia, sugar craving, headaches, aching joints, skin rashes , indigestion and perhaps an increased incidence of colds.

The following quote from Roger Williams who pioneered the concept of biochemical individuality is interesting:

'Some inbred rats on identical diets excreted 11 times as much urinary phosphate as others; some, when given a chance to exercise at will, ran consistently 20 times as far as others; some voluntarily consumed 16 times as much sugar as others; some drank 20 times as much alcohol; some appeared to need about 40 times as much vitamin A as others; some young guinea pigs required, for good growth, at least 20 times as much vitamin C as others.'

Human beings also have a range of biochemical individuality[3], which means that deficiencies may present themselves in different ways and with different underlying deficiency needs. The RDA levels may be

3   Williams RJ & Pelton RB. Individuality in
     Nutrition.Proc.N.A.C 1966;55:126

totally inadequate for that particular patient and Integrative doctors often find that very much higher doses are required for some people. Orthomolecular medicine is the use of high dose of certain nutrients. Vitamin C, Vitamin B3 (niacin), vitamin A, folate and many other nutrients may be used in very high doses in order to overcome the deficient needs of certain individuals

All chronic disease will have a background of some nutrient deficiencies. Keep in mind the following facts:

- Vitamin D: possibly 80% deficient in most populations. I very seldom see someone with normal levels of vitamin D. Perhaps we have all been frightened into spending too little time in the sun.

- Vitamin C: Some scientists like Linus Pauling, the Nobel Laureate believe that we need doses much higher than the RDA, which is about 60mg/day. His suggested intake is just below bowel tolerance, which may be between 3 to 10 g per day. In one American survey 26% of the population consumed less than 70% of the RDA. The elderly, smokers and institutionalised individuals are at a much greater risk of deficiency in vitamin C due to poor quality food, overcooked food and poor storage. The elderly are also seriously deficient in vitamin D.

- Vitamin A: 31% of USA population consumes less than 2/3 of the RDA and deficiency causes a profound disturbance of the immune system. Deficiency of this vitamin also causes serious eye problems in many parts of Africa.

- Vitamin Bs: Widespread deficiencies and poor intake because of refining of grains. Folic acid deficiencies for example are extremely common. In the USA the average intake is half of the RDA.

- Magnesium: 40% deficiency in many populations

- Selenium: 30% deficient and even more so in countries where the soil is seriously deficient in this mineral.

- Zinc: major deficiencies in zinc. One survey found that 68% of all adults consumed less than 2/3 of the RDA for zinc.

- Iodine: major deficiencies. This is so serious that iodine is added to salt (iodized salt) and even bread. Iodine is not only essential for thyroid hormone production but also required by breast and prostate. Consider the fact that under activity of the thyroid is epidemic and that breast and prostate cancer are two major problems we see today. This does not mean that iodine deficiency is the cause of these problems. Very few diseases have a single underlying cause but certainly iodine deficiency could be an important contributing causal factor.

Nutrient deficiencies may include vitamins, minerals, trace minerals, amino acids, essential fatty acids, fibre, simple carbohydrates and a range of other nutrients, some which the body can make and some which it cannot.

Nutrient deficiencies are present in everyone and will affect the function of many systems and even the way the body responds to drugs.

e: Mental-Emotional-Spiritual Equilibrium

Throughout this book I refer to the mind-body connection and while doctors tend to be dismissive of this connection as a contributing cause of serious diseases like cancer, Parkinson's disease, multiple sclerosis, SLE etc. this lack of interest makes no sense if one only spends a little time thinking about it.

Thought can make the hand go up, head turn, blood pressure go up, heart go faster, butterfly's in the stomach, even faint at the sight of a needle, vomit when confronted by something disgusting etc. When some emotion is buried in consciousness then its physiological arm is still active. The emotion has not gone away and can be activated by a thousand stimuli, in this way the physiological pressure is also just below the surface until eventually physical symptoms and signs begin to manifest which can eventually over many years lead to disease.

All diseases have a range of unconscious triggers, many buried in the unconscious since childhood often rising to the surface but more often just below the surface setting off little fires with physiological components that over time disrupt and stress that natural harmonious flow of physiological processes.

Mind is soaked into the body and its manifestations can be seen in the eyes and body language.

f: Organ Balance

Medical specialists are categorised according to the particular body organ they specialise in, such as cardiologists who specialise in heart and vascular problems, gastroenterologists who specialise in the gastrointestinal tract, nephrologists who specialise in kidney diseases, urologists who specialise is prostate and bladder problems etc. These specialists know more and more about their particular speciality and lose track over time of this particular organs connection to the rest of the body's systems.

Chinese Traditional Medicine (TCM) taught me that all the various systems of the body functioned together and that any disturbance of the one system has an effect on other systems that 'help' compensate and maintain the overall homeostasis. The way that TCM keeps the idea of 'wholeness' together is the recognition that we are always dealing with 'systems' and not organs. That organ damage is really the 'end point' of a system which has malfunctioned for a long time.

In the conventional medical model there is no clear idea of 'system dysfunction' but instead by developing a model based on 'parts' rather than systems and 'pathology' rather than 'functional integrity' specialists have focused on the physical organ and then treat that physical organ as a part, which is broken. This may mean removing the damaged organ and replacing it with another organ, removing the part of the organ diseases or damaged or using powerful drugs to block pain or treat inflammation.

Without a sense of the whole system however, treating the organ in isolation as if the rest of the body systems are disconnected with what is going on and are not already doing their best to keep control of the whole, is very reductionistic thinking.

The moment one recognises that the body functions as a whole unified system and not as isolated organs then suddenly there is the possibility of understand why the simplest approaches used by all traditional systems to treating any condition in the body, is to do a simple water or a vegetable juice fast. Such a simple fast allows the whole system to deal with the problematic areas that are manifesting as a dysfunctional organ.

The organ itself does not always have to be treated as a problem. It is the system as a whole that is stressed and the stress taking lines of least resistance ends up as an organ problem. Treating the organ without correcting the underlying dysfunction as indicated over and over again in this book is doing a disservice to the patient.

The organs are part of operating systems with extensions throughout the body and make up the matter-energy- informational web of activity.

g: Electro-magnetic Health

I have written a whole chapter on 'energy medicine' (Chapter 13) and only wish to point out again the recognition that Integrative doctors give to 'energy' with regard to health and ill health. Every condition must have an electro-magnetic component to it because a human being is not just a body but matter-energy -information system.

The ECG recording of the heart for example can be detected throughout the body with each heartbeat. This complex wave must have some influence on every cell of the body. Radiation can cause serious harm and even stimulate carcinogenic changes in the body. There is increasing evidence that cell phones can also harm. Magnetic fields can pass right through the body and our understanding of the subtle influence of all these fields of energy on the body is still in its infancy.

Electro-magnetic pollution is regarded as a serious problem by many scientists. Other scientists merely point to the fact that there is not enough evidence that electromagnetic influences can cause ill health.

Clearly people listen to who they want to hear and either pay attention to those who warn about electro-magnetic pollution or agree that there is not enough scientific evidence. I would be very cautious about dismissing the warning. All of life has developed within electromagnetic fields.

There is evidence for example that microwaves from cell phones can damage DNA and the International Agency for Research on Cancer (IARC) has classified ELF (extremely low frequency microwaves) and RF EMFs (Radio Frequency microwaves) as possibly carcinogenic to humans.

We are dealing with many subtle frequencies and waves without much science to support or dispute the assertion of some scientists, nevertheless common sense should warn us not to dismiss the possibility that electromagnetic energy in all its many manifestations could cause health but could also cause ill health. These energies are used throughout the world to heal and clearly the ECG and EEG have physiological effects in the body. We should not be surprised therefore that there is also a negative side to 'energy'.

Energy – information could be the next field of interest and research for medical progress moving beyond chemistry.

h: Cell Membrane Health

Integrative doctors are particularly concerned about cell membrane health. The cell is almost a living system in its own right. It protects those important structures, the DNA and RNA, from mutations and contains within its membranes also the mitochondria producing the energy bundles required for all functions in the body.

The cell membrane is astonishing in its ability to sense exactly what is required to maintain the internal environment of the cell, remove toxins, absorb the many nutrients necessary not only to feed the various functional 'bodies' within its borders and defend those structures from serious attacks by free radicals, viruses, bacteria, parasites and toxic chemicals.

There are 30 trillion cells in the human body with thousands of these cells dying and being replicated. All this requires nutrients and perhaps the most essential nutrients for membrane health are the fatty acids in the correct proportions.

The cell membrane is an active participant in homeostasis, maintaining a healthy balance within the cell and protecting the inner organelles from the outer cellular environment.

i: Mitochondrial Health

Mitochondria are tiny organs within each cell functioning like tiny generators of energy. They are probably the most active little organelles within the body constantly churning out ATP energy. Just like a coal engine needing huge amounts of coal to generate the power needed to drive the engine, mitochondria use huge amounts of nutrients to produce the ATP. This includes coenzyme Q10, L-carnitine, D-ribose.

Statins interestingly enough not only block the production of cholesterol but also coenzyme Q10. Using statins to prevent heart disease seems strange when one considers that the organ with the highest concentration of mitochondria is the heart muscle. They need a constant 24-hour supply of ATP energy. Coenzyme Q10 is essential to this function which statins block. Makes no sense unless statins were combined with coenzyme Q10. That for some very strange reason is not done.

Mitochondria are the powerhouse for energy and need a constant supply of nutrients.

j: Hypothalamic-Pituitary-Adrenal/ Thyroid/Ovaries/Testes Axis Balance

The hypothalamus is one of the most important hormonal glands positioned within the brain. On a slightly deeper level is the Thalamus, which is part of the brain. The hypothalamus controls the pituitary also positioned within the brain and this gland controls the adrenals, thyroid, testes and ovaries. The controls are on a feedback loop so that the glands are constantly feeding back information to each other in order to maintain homeostasis/balance.

It is via this link that brain activity can also influence hormonal functions, that stress can influence menstrual cycles, interest in sex, disturb gastro-intestinal motility, cause adrenal stress and thyroid disturbances. Treating the end organ again without paying attention to the chronic underlying stress, which works its way via the hypothalamic- pituitary- glandular axis, is not supporting health but treating the disease.

In my experience the emotional-mental stresses are often the most important causes, not only in such conditions as chronic fatigue, headaches and indigestion but also more serious conditions such as endometriosis, asthma, heart disease but even cancer. There are few diseases where stress does not play a significant role in the underlying cause but also in the eventual outcome of the condition.

Stress is both a significant cause of most ill health but also drives the eventual outcome.

k: Hormonal Health

Hormones are messengers spreading their influence throughout the body. There are hormones that surge into prominence during daily cycles like melatonin which is active at night, inducing sleep and other hormones with monthly cycles like oestrogen and progesterone. Other hormones are swinging up and down depending on the physiological needs such as insulin (dependent on food eaten), adrenalin, cortisone (dependent on level of emotional and physical stress) and thyroid hormones (dependent on metabolic requirements).

Hormones don't function in isolation, which means that with the rhythmic cycles a whole range of other physiological functions must also adjust to this rhythm. Any disturbance of these rhythms also means pressure on other systems to help maintain the best balance possible.

During the life span of each person there are major adjustments required as children reach puberty, mature sexually, move onto menopause/andropause and then grow old over time. These adjustments involve the whole body and may be more or less stressful resulting in no symptoms if the system is fluid and adaptable; or if the system is rigid and deficient in its ability to make these major shifts there will be various symptoms of change.

Menopause in women is a classic time for stress within the system causing more or less discomfort as the hormones fall. This decline can follow many different patterns. What is required during this time, are not always more hormones, as the fall in hormones is a natural process and many women go through menopause without symptoms.

Generally symptoms are due to the fact that progesterone falls much faster than the oestrogen leading to what is described as relative oestrogen dominance. While giving bio-identical progesterone will often help this condition, Integrative practitioners have also learnt that by just maximising nutrients, changing lifestyle with better food choices, removing sugar from the diet, exercise and stress management will all improve symptoms and signs. This is the classic approach of supporting general health rather than just treating the condition.

Just supporting and trying to optimise health can influence hormonal function.

1: Drugs Interfering with Function

Please check out chapter 16 Drugs vs. Natural products and how they differ in functions and the way they are used. Anti-histamines, beta blockers, serotonin reuptake inhibitors, proton pump inhibitors give a very clear indication of what these drugs do and why they require really strict guidelines in use, serious research in laboratories, animal models and finally human trials, first with volunteers and then the public domain which is the final 'great experiment'.

One needs to be very clear that even when the drug is finally released into the public domain, they are not exactly safe. Drugs are always only relatively safe for the simple reason that they work by interfering with a function and can therefore always have potential side effects.

Drugs interfere with function therefore increase the dysfunction within the system and cause side effects.

m: Gastrointestinal Health

Essential to the functional integrity of the body is the gastrointestinal tract, which is responsible for taking the food ingested and breaking it down into its smallest molecules that can be absorbed through the mucous membrane. It is an astonishing process. Food which is contaminated with micro-organism and parasites must be made safe for absorption. The stomach acid is so strong that little can survive in its passage through this organ and yet this same acid must be neutralised in the small intestine very rapidly in order to allow the enzymes from the pancreas to function.

These enzymes require an alkaline medium. So the food passes from a seriously acidic environment in the stomach and is then held long enough in that environment by the pyloric valve, the gatekeeper from the stomach to the duodenum. It then must pass into the alkaline medium due to the secretions of the pancreas which also contain the enzymes for further digestion and with bile added to this mix from the gall bladder.

The seriously acidic fluid in the physiological mechanisms are precise and the controls underlying this process appear to be in touch with the whole digestive process.

Proton pump inhibitors which block acid secretion and seem to decrease heartburn may make clinical sense but clearly place shackles on the precision required to maintain a normal balance of the physiological process required for the whole digestive tract.

The Integrative way is to work at changing the diet, decrease the stress which interferes with acid control, use herbs which help normal physiological modulation of acid secretion, lift the head of the bed so that acids no longer flow up into the oesophagus at night and support the digestive process with additional enzymes or bile.

Beyond the stomach is the duodenum where the pancreatic secretions enter together with bile and liver secretions to continue the digestive process. All these functions require enormous amount of energy, nutrients to produce the energy, cofactors for enzyme functions, litres of bicarbonate containing fluid to alkalinise the acid secretions pouring in from the stomach. The pancreas produces about 8 cups of liquid secretions per day. The intestines also secrete mucous to protect the lining with enormous capacity to absorb the broken down food components.

Perhaps this gives some idea of the activity going on in the intestinal tract and why again good food choices are required. Junk food, processed foods will not provide the body with all the nutrients required for the constant and life long need to digest and absorb and provide the energy to make this possible.

Try to keep in mind that like all processes happening right across the functioning processes of the body, cell membranes, mitochondria, pH control, hormone balance , liver function etc all need to be co-ordinated for everything else to function well.

Digestion of food and absorption of nutrients is a complex day and night activity drawing on a constant need of good quality food to maintain healthy functions.

n: Sleep

So much happens during the sleep state that it is surprising how little attention doctors pay to sleep patterns. It is mainly during sleep that the body recuperates from the energy expenditure of the day. Everyone eventually becomes exhausted and needs to lie down and sleep for hours. I personally am a catnapper and for as long as I can remember need to have 10 to 30 minute naps between 1 and 2 pm whether I eat or don't eat. A cup of coffee in the morning can sometimes shift me past this low point.

That short nap makes all the difference to my afternoon. So something quite dramatic and profound happens during sleep. During the day energy stored is used up and the body systems slowly run down while at night during the sleep state the physical body is 're-tuned', the energy deficit made up again and one generally feels ready for another day when waking up in the morning. This is a remarkable process and little understood.

During sleep the thinking mind stops functioning and waking consciousness is no longer present. Body functions continue, suggesting that the waking consciousness and thinking mind need to be shut down for the re-tuning process to happen. Sleep is obviously an important healing modality required for optimum health.

Is therefore taking conventional synthetic sleeping pills a good idea?

Drugs work by interfering or blocking a biochemical process. As Breggin[4], the psychiatrist has pointed out many times... '"*All drugs that impact on the brain and mind 'work' by partially disabling the brain and mind. No psychoactive substance corrects biochemical imbalances or any other real and presumed defects, deficits or disorders of the brain and mind, and none improve the function of the brain and mind. The so-called therapeutic effect is always a disability.*'

As he points out, drugs do not have the specific effects as claimed by their name e.g. anxiolytic or hypnotics but work instead by depressing brain function in a more general way in which a specific effect may sometimes be dominant amongst a range of other depressive effects.

The sleep pattern has an intrinsic rhythm to it, which is in synchronicity with a range of functions in the body. The 'retuning' process is not just happening in the head but involves every organ and process in the body. It requires a unique kind of sensitivity, feedback information and a return to coherence that involved not just biochemistry but energy and information.

Drugs cannot induce a normal sleep. Daniel F Kripke MD, professor of psychiatry at the University of California, worked for 30 years assessing the risk of sleeping pills. His findings were stunning and showed that people who take sleeping pills die sooner than people who do not (British Medical Journal February 2012). Sleeping pills he said may have been associated with 320,000 to 507,000 excess deaths in the USA alone. Sleeping pill users also had a 35 % higher risk of cancer. Clearly taking sleeping pills interferes with the normal sleep rhythm and prevents a healthy 're-tuning' of the body.

During normal sleep, healing, detoxification and energy build-up occurs preparing the body for the next day's activity.

4   Breggin PR Rational Principles of Psychopharm- acology for Therapists, Healthcare Providers and Clients. J Contemp Psychother 2016; 46:1-13

o: Anti-Oxidant/Free Radical Balance

Antioxidants and free radicals are polar opposites but each essential to maintaining a balance within the body. The free radicals have one less electron in their orbit and run around looking for another electron to fill into that space. This makes them extremely aggressive and even destructive.

In Chinese Traditional terminology, they are 'yang', have a masculine characteristic, operate in bands of aggressive molecules sweeping through the body spaces killing micro-organism which is good but also can kill and destroy normal cells standing in their way.

They can damage DNA, damage mitochondria and set the stage for serious disease manifesting. Stress, smoking, many processed foods, pollution, nuclear radiation can all generate free radicals. No chronic disease has a single underlying cause and free radical damage is one of the causes present in most ill health.

Anti-oxidants on the other hand are 'yin', feminine in character, supportive and nourishing, holding back the onrush of the free radicals by providing them with the electron that they need to satisfy their lust. It is why so many natural foods are healthy for us as they contain a good supply of anti-oxidants.

Antioxidants protect body from excess destruction of free radicals

p: Good Hydration

It is important to maintain good hydration. Half the body weight is water and water is the background for every process within the body. Each persons needs are different so it is important to be aware of drinking liquid that is not sugar saturated. Herb teas are a fine way to drink water and these can easily be drunk without adding a sweetener. Most of my liquid intake comes from green tea with added water if I am exercising, in the sauna or in hot weather and sweating. I can usually tell when I am not drinking sufficient liquid by the colour of my urine. If it is too yellow then I have not been drinking enough water.

Keep urine light in colour by drinking adequate water.

q: Acid-Alkaline Balance

The body maintains a very tight control of the acid-alkaline balance so that the food one eats does not make major changes in that balance, but can stress this balance towards the acid or alkaline side of the equation.

With the different diets recommended e.g. the more acid forming protein, fat diet compared to a more alkaline vegetarian diet it is not surprising that many of us get quite confused. I have watched in surprise at the way friends of mine changing to the high fat, protein and low carbohydrate diet which I would normally regard as acid forming tell me how much better they feel, weight reduced and many symptoms of ill health disappear.

While cancer is said to thrive in an acid environment I remember a patient with breast cancer who despite a year on a raw food very alkaline diet had no improvement in her breast cancer and eventually had increasing spread of the cancer. On the other hand the high fat, moderate protein and low carbohydrate diet is used to treat a number of cancers particularly brain cancer and will control many children with epilepsy.

Aging is said to be associated with an increasingly acid environment leading to death eventually of cells and increasing cancerous tissue. So I can understand the confusion around firstly choosing the right diet and relating health to the acid-alkaline environment. Perhaps the answer to this dilemma lies again in the biochemical uniqueness of each person and that there is no one diet that fits everyone and that some individuals operate better on the more acid than the alkaline side of the divide. Be careful of allowing the thinking mind make the decision. Allow the feeling and intuitive self to also be part of the decision committee and check it out for yourself.

Each person has a unique biochemical profile requiring unique diet to produce the unique acid-alkaline balance required by the body for healthy function.

r: Stomach Acid Normal

The stomach is an incredible organ. It secretes an acid strong enough to corrode metal and at the same time has an exquisite control over this process secreting protective mucus preventing the acid from eating into the tissues. If the acid secretion is too high however or the mucus lining is insufficient then the acid will irritate the mucous membrane and cause inflammation.

Nevertheless the resilience of the lining always astonishes me and the fact that ulceration is less common than it is and that the acid does not eat its way all through the stomach lining attests to the full array of protective mechanisms still present even when ulceration is present.

The many roles of acid secretion in the stomach

• To maintain a sterile environment in the stomach and prevent the contamination of small bowel with micro-organism.

• To initiate the conversion of pepsinogen to pepsin required for the digestion of protein.

• Acid dumped into the duodenum stimulates the release of gastric inhibitory peptide, secretin (effects pancreatic function) and cholecystokinin (effects gall bladder function) from the duodenum. Disruption of this process may cause disorders of digestion in the small intestine.

• Acid and pepsin is a prerequisite for optimum digestion.

• Acidic pH also has an important influence on the absorption of selected micronutrients especially minerals such as calcium, magnesium and Zinc and also vitamins such as folic acid, ascorbic acid and beta-carotene. Zinc solubility for example is dependent on pH with increasing solubility occurring as the pH becomes more acidic.

• There is some correlation between low acid secretion and a range of medical conditions such as chronic skin conditions, digestive disturbances, alcoholism, and intestinal permeability, overgrowth of pathological bacteria, fungi and parasites. All these conditions may benefit from hydrochloric acid supplementation.

Despite the importance of stomach acid to protect the body from contamination from the external environment in the food consumed and to digest protein, medical doctors often prescribe acid blocking agents (PPPIs) to lower the acid secretion and treat heartburn and acid reflux. While this will work short term it all to often becomes a chronic prescription.

This clearly cannot be healthy for the body and other more natural prescription and approaches are available. These include raising the head of the bed to prevent reflux at night with one brick, mastic gum, probiotics, Siberian pine nut oil and decreasing sugar and grains from the diet. The latter dietary changes may in fact make all the difference.

Right stomach acid concentration is key to digestion and maintaining a sterile environment.

s: Inflammation Control

Inflammation is a normal and natural response to injury whether it is a fall or a surgical knife cutting tissue or damage due to invading micro-organisms. It is the way the body heals itself. It is a protective response involving many cells and tissues and has as its goals the removal of the initial cause of tissue injury if possible, to remove the damaged tissue and finally to repair the damage done.

The inflammatory response contains all the ingredients that the body needs to heal under normal and acute conditions. It is when this process continuous over the long term that the same elements used to heal can also cause serious disturbance and the inflammatory response then becomes self destructive.

The inflammatory soup contains free radicals, toxic chemicals that need constant removing by components from the blood and surrounding tissue which make up the immune system response to injury and what is required to heal. The same components however used to destroy micro-organism can also damage normal tissue. This means that very tight control is required that can become out of control if the inflammatory process is excessive or the controls are inadequate.

Chronic inflammation can be self-destructive.

Conclusion

There are many regulatory processes in the body required to maintain balance and homeostasis. I have mentioned quite a few of them in the above discussion, nevertheless these are only a small part of the myriad processes happening in every moment of time. There are many other biochemical dysfunctions possible, DNA distortions and unique individual variations, a range of emotional-mental attitudes and stress unique to that person, a range of different nutritional deficiencies and unique needs for that individual.

The totality of these dysfunction set up patterns of disturbances that slowly or rapidly take lines of least resistance towards increasing dysfunction causing signs and symptoms that eventually end up as disease patterns that are recognised and diagnosed as a disease entity. While the process may sometimes be rapid, generally it can take many years to end up with the 'disease'.

During the intermediate years the person will have a range of many different appearances of ill health including various gastro-intestinal symptoms, recurrent colds or flues, recurrent headaches or migraine, periods of extreme tiredness and fuzzy head, swelling of the legs, aches and pains around the body. Symptoms will come and go as the body manages to adjust to the stresses and strains. Often just making small changes to diet, resting a little more, letting go of stressful situations, going on holiday is enough to help the body cope better.

As I emphasise many times in this book, the body has a natural innate healing mechanism that is always correcting any dysfunction. If healing is not happening in that moment it is only because the systems in the body are not coping. Integrative doctors understand that it is not necessary to fill up all the holes, to correct every deficiency or remove every stress factor to initiate a healing response.

The body wants to heal and often just a little support in a few places can make all the difference. Tiredness disappears, headaches dissolve and the indigestion smooth's itself away. This is the body at work, doing what it knows well enough to do. Natural medicine can support the process. Drugs block functions, which may help in a symptomatic way in the short term but may also prevent the innate healing process from doing its natural work.

Chapter 15

The rare but spectacular phenomenon of spontaneous remission of cancer persists in the annals of medicine, totally inexplicable but real, a hypothetical straw to clutch in the search for cure. From time to time patients turn up with far advanced cancer, beyond the possibility of cure. They undergo exploratory surgery, the surgeon observes metastases throughout the peritoneal cavity and liver, and the patient is sent home to die, only to turn up again 10 years later free of disease and in good health. There are now several hundred such cases in world scientific literature, and no one doubts the validity of the observations.

But no one has the ghost of an idea how it happens.'[1]

Spontaneous Remissions

Spontaneous remissions, the placebo response, the power of prayer and even mind over matter healing fall into the same category of healing and give some insight into a process that happens so naturally that it tends to get dismissed as woo woo medicine, folk medicine, miracles of no special interest and certainly nothing to do with 'real medicine'.

I have always found this very strange. Why would any healing that is not invasive, happens spontaneously in a very creative way, does not even require much effort, be ignored by the medical profession.

Clearly it does not follow medical protocol, can't be subjected to conventional medical science and tends to be dismissed by medical doctors who follow a different reality of medicine in which miraculous healing appears to be so rare that it can be ignored as inconsequential and not important to the larger problem of dealing with chronic disease.

As indicated in the chapter on the placebo response the rarity of this kind of healing should be questioned. In fact it is so common that no drug trial can be done without a placebo arm. While the focus of everyone is on the drug response, the fact is that the placebo response has always intrigued

---

1   Lewis Thomas, The Youngest Science: Notes of a
      Medical Watcher(Viking Press 1983,205)

me and I have wondered how many drug trials have not been published because the placebo has actually done much better than the drug.

These are regarded as negative studies i.e. the placebo arm suggest that the drug is no more effective than the placebo. Scientists and their pharmaceutical backers don't like to publish these studies and will just repeat the study making slight adjustments until better results are obtained. Better results mean that the drug does better than the placebo.

Is there a difference between spontaneous healing , the power of prayer and the placebo response. I don't think that in principle they are different responses, so in this chapter we will tease this open and investigate why I think so and how it actually works in the real world of physiology.

In 'Spontaneous Remissions' an annotated bibliography from the Institute of Noetic Sciences they have the following definition of spontaneous remissions:

'The disappearance, complete or incomplete, of a disease or cancer without medical treatment or treatment that is considered inadequate to produce the resulting disappearance of disease symptoms or tumour'.

This definition could just as easily apply to the 'placebo response' or even the response to prayer.

There appears to me to be some clear logic in the process of healing as I have tried to clarify in this book.

The body has its own innate healing potential and mechanisms in place.

I have over and over again referred to this innate healing ability which is normal and natural and miraculous only in the sense that it is so complex that it is difficult to even comprehend how this could take place from moment to moment.

We know the maps and any text book of physiology or biochemistry discusses these maps i.e. the description of the classic process. Nevertheless the actual way each unique person's physiology functions is still a mystery and astonishingly complex. There are very good reasons for this. The following factors account for the variability and why text book explenations are only generalised maps and not the territory of each unique person:

- Genetic variability (e.g. folic acid) and genetic variations account for the fact that People may Vary Enormously in their quantitative need for this essential vitamin.

- People eat different diets which contain toxins, variable amounts of nutrients and cofactors required for physiological function

- People have different chronic emotional streams of reactions effecting the way the body functions

- We are all affected differently by the background electro-magnetic noise and gravitational fields which surround us.

- The genetic variability, the toxic load in the environment plus emotional stress together with many other environmental factors move the dysfunctional process along lines of least resistance towards its breakdown (the disease).

Doctors not focused on the diseased end point but who are able to step back as it were, notice that each person is unique in how they express the inner disturbances as physiological problems and have learnt the following:

- The system functions holistically. A system is a system is a system. Systems cannot be broken apart. They can be teased open but the moment we cut and break the system, it must either re-orientate into another functioning system or it just stops working.

- The system is intelligent. There is so much happening in every moment of time that it requires more than just feedback systems to operate. There must be an overall intelligence holding everything together.

- Healing is constantly at work to maintain homeostasis . Healing or health maintenance is what the system does well and is built into every part of its fibre.

- The ill health and disease is the best the body can do under the circumstances. The whole system is always doing the best it can do. Any dysfunction within the system is still under control and the best the system can do.

- Only the system can heal itself given the right circumstance. Healing belongs to the system. It is innate right down to the smallest detail. Any other addition is merely supportive.

What does all this actually say about the human system as a whole and especially about its capacity to heal itself in terms of what we know today .

Some important questions come up:

- Where is this intelligence situated

- Why does the system malfunction if it is so intelligent

- What is actually happening within the system as it moves towards disease

Where are the controls within the body?

Most doctors don't bother themselves with this question and are generally dismissive of such questions from patients, by suggesting that the controls are all in the brain, despite the fact that there is no evidence that this is so.

Nevertheless this is an important question to ask . We will see very shortly that the answer is not at all straight forward and may point us in a direction that right now may have no definitive answer .

Clearly there must be very exquisite controls that keep so many functions operating at such a precise and fine level. Consider how precise the temperature of the body is maintained despite enormous variation in outside body conditions from people living in steaming hot jungle conditions to dry hot desert conditions to freezing temperatures far below those conditions that most living systems are able to thrive in. When a person develops a fever this very fine control is still maintained as the temperature rises and reaches a plateau that is seldom crossed as the very life of the organism may be threatened above a certain level.

The body has both clotting and anticlotting mechanisms which again are finely controlled preventing excessive bleeding or clotting within the blood vessels. The sympathetic and parasympathetic nervous system are again finely tuned so that neither dominates for prolonged periods.The two systems control each other providing the exact mix required for fight and flight mechanisms, contraction and relaxation, stimulation and sedation. Feedback systems are everywhere, preventing any activity from dominating for prolonged periods.

Imagine the control required for digestion, the exact amount of hydrochloric acid, enough mucous lining the stomach to prevent the acid from digesting the stomach itself, enough acid to breakdown the protein in the meal, sufficient bicarbonate to neutralise the acid pouring into the duodenum and creating the exact conditions so that the enzymes secreted by the pancreas can function within their optimum range.

The acid from the stomach flowing into the duodenum however is also essential to keep the upper digestive tract free of micro-organism which is so plentiful in the lower bowel. So precise and beautifully co-ordinated are these processes in order to breakdown the food into the particles required for absorption.

Apart from these more obvious levels of control, there are much finer levels of control down at the cellular level allowing and preventing a range of chemicals from passing into and out-of each cell. Magnesium for example is required inside the cell while sodium is mainly outside the cell.

Even within each cell there are minute intracellular organs such as the mitochondria, golgi body etc which also have membranes that control the passage of nutrients in and out. The mitochondria produce energy and require oxygen and nutrients in very definite amounts and balance for physiological functions elsewhere.

All of this has to be very tightly controlled and balanced with other systems and environments within the body.

Imagine the opening ceremony of an Olympic games with thousands of people taking part, plus the music team, props team, singers, dancers, light technicians etc. All this has to be co-ordinated and rehearsed over and over again. That is the easy part but what happens if there is a blackout in the middle of the show, or the lead singer collapses, or a fire breaks out that spreads rapidly, chaos would most likely occur but in the body the intelligence co-ordinating function is still able to deal with most challenges.

In order to do this it must have contact with what is happening all over the body on a moment to moment basis. We are talking about trillions of processes with a very fine window within which it must operate.

As Bill Bryson describes it in 'A Short History of Nearly Everything':

'If you could visit a cell, you wouldn't like it. Blown up to a scale at which atoms were about the size of peas, a cell itself would be a sphere roughly half a mile across, and supported by a complex framework of

girders called a cytoskeleton. Within it, millions upon millions of objects – some the size of basketballs, others the size of cars – would whiz about like bullets. There wouldn't be a place you could stand without being pummelled and ripped thousands of times every second from every direction. Even for its full-time occupants the inside of a cell is a hazardous place. Each strand of DNA is on average attacked or damaged once every 8.4 seconds – ten thousand times in a day- by chemicals and other agents that whack into or carelessly slice through it, and each of these wounds must be swiftly stitched up if the cell is not to perish.'

If this is happening in every cell of the body and all has to be co-ordinated within fractions of a moment then where could those controls be, when the movement of chemicals and chemical messengers around the body are much too slow to make this possible.

If we return to our 'greater anatomy' story then it is possible to turn to the 'energy-information' aspects of the greater anatomy. Matter/biochemistry is not going to give us an answer to this problem. We need to look elsewhere!

Energy-information certainly moves at much greater speed and moves easily through matter. Magnetic fields for example penetrate matter almost as if no matter is present. Iron filings will fall into place around a magnet and get dragged around by a moving magnetic field. Energy carries information or information flows along electromagnetic fields. The picture on the TV screen is dependent on the copper wire, the electricity flowing along the wire and the information carried by the electricity.

The human body is run through with a range of electromagnetic fields such as the electromagnetic field of the heart, the ECG and the EEG which is the electromagnetic field of the brain, but there are also a range of other fields within and around as well. The magnetic field of the earth can move the oceans so that one should not be surprised that the same field can influence biochemistry and why astronauts flying into outer space away from the influence of the earths magnetic field must be enclosed within a magnetic field inside their capsule.

The speed of electromagnetic signals is 300 000 kilometres per second, while the speed of a diffusible chemical is only in the range of 1 centimetre per second. The latter speed would never be able to meet the needs of a system shifting its requirements from moment to moment.

In Traditional Chinese Medicine the heart is said to be the 'Emperor' controlling the whole kingdom. Not surprising then that doctors measure the electromagnetic field of the heart by placing electrodes on the wrist, ankles and over the heart. This complex wave of the heart field moves rapidly all over the body penetrating every cell to the tips of the fingers and toes and to the top of the head, moving through every organ and cell of the body. If energy carries information then one may wonder what messages are being sent by the Emperor to the rest of the kingdom.

If the controls are vested in the energy-information realm then is there still a deeper level of control? Who or what controls the energy-information. Strangly enough science is already pointing to an answer, so lets just have a look how quantum science and in particular the work of David Bohm is helping to understand where the controls could be.

If we examine the nature of an atom, keeping in mind along the way that all of matter is made of atoms, then we come across the reality that most of matter is empty space with 'particles' appearing and disappearing back into that surrounding space. Particles cant exactly be captured apart from their imprint on a photographic plate because they appear and disappear in fractions of seconds. The reality is that the so called objects or your body for example is made of atoms which are made of particles that appear and disappear throwing out energy in very discrete ways and there is a lot of empty space all around.

This empty space was once thought to be really empty, like a vacuum with no 'stuff' in it. Scientists are re-looking at this empty space and discovering to their amazement that actually it is not empty but full of potential. David Bohm calls this the 'quantum potential' and it is the deepest level that scientists can agree on. At this level there is no 'stuff' but everything and all stuff seems to emerge out of this vast limitless space of potential.

If all the 'stuff' of matter appears out of the quantum potential in such an ordered way so that there is no apparent chaos in this emerging i.e. all the stuff of matter appears and disappears almost as fast as it appears and yet maintains the structure in its original form, then there must be some control element within the quantum potential.

Now what could that be?

This is a great mystery. Is it possible that the controls present in this quantum potential could contain the controls for every living organism in the world, for reconstructing every 'matter' object made of atoms which contain particles appearing and disappearing. The ancients in every continent thought so.

Later there was the supreme God in control and now science and many scientists have come to believe that this God lives in the quantum space guiding the movement at the most fundamental level of all particles, making the 'stuff' of the universe. What name you call this 'control system' is really not important but there is an increasing agreement that all the names refer to the same thing. Some people call this God, others call it the quantum potential, Great Mystery, All Encompassing Abyss, Infinity etc.

The characteristics of this agreement is that what is being referred to is present everywhere, appears all powerful in the sense that it is controls, directs and appears to be the creative edge of all 'matter' on earth and it appears to be in contact with everything at the same time.

The heart-brain connection.

In their introduction to their book on the heart, the Heart Math Institute says the following:

'New research shows the human heart is much more than an efficient pump that sustains life. Our research suggests the heart also is an access point to a source of wisdom and intelligence that we can call upon to live our lives with more balance, greater creativity and enhanced intuitive capacities. All of these are important for increasing personal effectiveness, improving health and relationships and achieving greater fulfillment.'

The Heart Math Institute is at the frontier of amazing research especially with regard to understanding the 'heart' as much more than just a pump, but rather as an intelligent and creative centre of activity. In Traditional Chinese medicine all the organs of the body are creative intelligences.

Again this is not referring to the anatomical material organ only but the 'Orb' understanding in which the material organ is just an anchor of a much larger dimensional intelligence. In the same way that the human being is not just a body but a body- emotions- mind-spirit being and matter-energy-information-consciousness being, so each organ also has a greater anatomy with an energy-informational aspect also connected to consciousness.

In the very reductionistic way of reducing human being to a body and then cells and physiology, it may appear that the hearts main function is pumping the blood around and yet when people are asked where their centre of 'feeling' is they tend to place their hand over their heart or sometimes over the abdomen when they refer to 'gut feeling'. Why is it that our experience of 'feeling' or even 'love' seems to emanate from the heart area.

This is what happens when there is a disconnect between scientific measurements, experience and theory. Scientific measurement is always limited and limiting. Experience and theory can work nicely together using scientific measurements to clarify, expand and enrich our understanding. Each has a place and neither alone will be enough to further our understanding of reality.

In Traditional Chinese Medicine the heart is not an organ but an 'Orb' with the heart organ functioning more as an anchor of the Orb. The heart Orb has a physical component, the organ itself plus an energetic/moving aspect and a nourishing supporting aspect. This is the Yin and Yang components of the heart. It is a functioning system of matter-energy-information.

What the Heart Math Institute has discovered is a very clear relationship between the heart and the brain and shows how theory and experience using science can enhance our understanding of the way life operates. By measuring the electromagnetic fields of the heart and brain, the coherence of these fields, i.e. the way these fields relate, support or disturb each other, the scientists of the Institute have discovered that the heart can affect our awareness, perception, intelligence and the way we respond in our daily life.

It seems, they say, that the 'heart has a mind of its own'. The more coherent the physiological state of the heart the increased emotional stability and resilience present in the system as a whole. They talk of the heart as a 'highly complex information- processing centre with its own functional brain, called the heart-brain that communicated with and influences brain activity via four pathways.' This includes neurological and biochemical communication systems, biophysical (pulse wave) and electromagnetic fields.

Research today has now reached a critical point requiring a major shift in the medical paradigm which is still very much stuck in the anatomical-biochemical model of health and ill health and where the diagnosis of disease as a 'matter problem' is no longer tenable based on the large volume of research now available. Using drugs which interfere with biochemistry and surgery and other invasive approaches which try and manipulate matter seems out of touch with what is already shifting in so many other areas of our lives.

Working with the control centre

Once it becomes clear that the control centre is not vested in the physical body but at the deeper level, and that even the electromagnetic fields within and around the body are also responding to a deeper level of control, then management of ill health and disease takes on a different perspective.

My viewpoint is that the controls are probably at the quantum level where instantaneous informational transfer can take place, and that ill health arises when the informational transfer is disturbed or blocked in some way. How then should health practitioners respond to such information. The answer turns out to be quite simple once the above is clearly defined:

- There is a deep seated control system maintaining harmony, coherence, equilibrium and homeostasis.

- This control system is in contact with every cell, every energy field, every molecule and right down to the atom.

- Ill health begins when interference factors in the outward flow of information along energy channels becomes such that it affects biochemistry eventually. This understanding is very close to that of many traditional healing systems but especially the TCM model in which the practitioners describe channels or meridians of energy flow and where disease arises when the energy becomes deficient, excessive or blocked.

- Once there is this understanding that the intelligence for healing is vested within the system at a deep quantum level then the health practitioner can develop a clear understanding of the management that is required to activate this innate self healing system.

- The placebo response, spontaneous healing, miraculous healing, power of prayer, hypnosis etc all point to the ability of this innate healing potential to co-ordinate a healing response beneficial to the whole organism.

Practitioners specialising in supporting health recognize then that any management protocol comes with the understanding that the system always has the potential to heal itself already in place. This potential has not gone anywhere. When this potential really does shut down then death of the body will occur.

Death may also occur if there are sufficient blocks in the system to prevent the innate healing potential from rising to the surface of physiological processes. The work of any health practitioner then is to remove the blocks which may be emotional blocks, toxic blocks, enzyme blocks etc and support and nourish physiological and energetic systems in the body .

Healing is a natural process going on all the time.

This is such an important statement and well recognised by most lay people and all health practitioners. It is why when we get a cold or 'flu or infectious disease we intrinsically know to just wait it out while the healing processes do their job of healing. Even surgeons recognize that after surgery everyone must wait for healing of the wound and tissues .

Sports injuries, middle ear infections in children, influenza, fractures of bones, menstrual bleeding, exhaustion at the end of the day, headaches, indigestion, food poisoning etc. will all disappear over time in the majority of cases just by resting and allowing this healing process to proceed.

Even when drugs are used, such as antibiotics, they do not in any way control or activate the healing processes. Antibiotics kill bacteria and this makes it easier for healing to happen. Drugs can reduce pain , interfere with the inflammatory process but the healing process is an innate intelligent process that will respond to support and nourishing.

As indicated elsewhere we are all exhausted, sleepy and even dysfunctional before going to sleep and under normal circumstances with a good nights sleep we wake up refreshed and ready for another day.

The complexity of this healing process is such that there needs to be constant feedback, very precise recognitions of the terrain conditions, the ability to call upon a range of nutrients, to activate enzymes in an exact way so that there is no waste of material. Energy from mitochondrial function (the generator of ATP energy) must be continuous, vitamin C is required in adequate amounts, the immune system must be vigilant and respond with the appropriate army of chemicals to heal and protect, the blood supply is required in exact amounts, oxygen is needed and whole range of other nutrients are required to make sure that the healing process flows towards healthy healing.

This enormous complexity is generally reduced to bite size pieces by textbooks, newspaper reports and by scientists trying to explain what is going on in living systems. Living systems do not work in linear mechanical ways in which a cause leads to an effect in a predictable outcome.

Even non-living systems in the real world cannot be said to be always perfectly predictable and this is why weather prediction remains and will always remain, just a prediction. The reason for this is that the smallest part within the system may spin itself into causing a transformative change that is unpredictable.

The butterfly effect in science states that the flapping of a butterfly wing in one part of the world can cause a storm in another part.

It is generally the 'missing information' that can make all the difference and there is always missing information in any investigation for the simple reason as indicated; the processes are so folded into each other and moving as such a speed that it is impossible to capture all the information or know how this information has been used by the system.

All this understanding is discussed today in the current terminology of quantum science under headings such as uncertainty principle, complementarity, chaos theory, wave-particle duality and the general idea that there are limits to what can be known and observed.

Scientists have begun to acknowledge something which the ancient philosopher Aristotle stated in one of his works written in the third century BC: 'It is the mark of an educated mind to rest satisfied with the degree of precision that the nature of the subject admits, and not to seek exactness when only an approximation is possible'[2]

Healing is therefore complex, is intrinsic and innate to the system, is controlled at a very deep level, deeper than physiology, reaching into the molecular-quantum level of the living organism. The recognition that the human system is matter-energy-information-quantum potential space and body-emotions-mind-spirit-consciousness suggests that the controls must be at the deepest level which is at the consciousness/quantum level. In a later chapter I will discuss how practitioners are beginning to understand how to work with this intelligence in a creative way.

2   Briggs J & Peat FD Turbulent Mirror.1990.Harper & Row p76

Chapter 16

The child had been crying all night. The parents noted a fever of 39 C with refusal to eat any food. She seemed dull and listless. It was decided to take the child to a pediatrician the next day who diagnosed a probably influenza or even an early stage of infectious disease. He prescribed some medication for pain and fever and another drug for inflammation.

The child continued to be unwell with a high fever all the next day and not eating. They telephoned the doctor who suggested they take an antibiotic just in case this was a bacterial infection. At this point the parents decided to come and see me.

On examination the fever was 38.5C. The eardrums looked normal. The throat was slightly red. No rash was present. Urine was clear and I suggested to the parents that this was most likely a viral infection such as Influenza. I stopped all the drugs which were clearly only symptomatic, told the parents to control the temperature with tepid sponging if necessary, make sure the child drank lots of water and take vitamin C two hourly with some homeopathic remedies for 'flu and high fever. I also added Echinaforce, a herbal remedy containing echinacea, an immune system adaptogen.

The child began to improve after 36 hours and made a good recovery.

Drugs vs Natural Products

There is a medical jargon used by both Integrative doctors and conventional medical doctors that is extremely confusing to everyone, especially patients who are recipients of 'medicines' from both kinds of doctors. Both groups of doctors use the same terminology but mean it in a very different way. What confounds the problem even more is that many medical doctors believe that they can use natural remedies 'to treat the disease' when this is not really the way most natural products work. As has been indicated many times in this book the Integrative approach to ill health is to support health rather than treat the disease.

Support health rather than treating the disease

This approach is absolutely fundamental to a holistic, natural and integrative management of ill health and separating out the difference between drugs and natural products. Using natural products to treat disease is nothing more than the conventional approach dressed up to look 'holistic' and 'natural'. Most natural medicines are not strong enough to work like drugs.

Calling natural products and drugs, 'medicines' is just another way to confuse the issue and leads people to believe that these two groups of products should be regulated in the same way within the same broad category and even classified according to the same group of conditions that they treat.

This is a serious error in thinking.

Are drugs and natural products 'medicines'?

The dictionary defines a 'medicine' as something which treats disease and can heal. This definition is problematic in my understanding as treating a disease and healing a person are really separate issues.

Treating a disease and healing a person

Integrative medicine and all traditional and natural healing systems focus on phase 1 (lifestyle) and phase 2 (the dysfunction) while medical doctors are trained to pay attention to phase 3 (the disease). The disease is the end point of many years of dysfunction driven by poor lifestyle habits and accumulation of toxins.

We know that cancer develops over many, many years and that behind the cancer are even more years of accumulated and increasing dysfunctions, which allow the cancer to slowly increase in size and sometimes spread.

By the time 'the disease' has manifested there is increasing dysfunctional processes throughout the body-mind system. Treating the disease only is like fixing the part that is broken in the motorcar without doing a tune-up and speaking to the driver. A good mechanic will do all three i.e. fix, tune and speak to the driver. Clearly fixing the part only and sending the car out without tuning and speaking to the driver is a very poor job indeed.

Drugs modify one or more of the functions of living systems by interfering with that function.

This modification process results in a change to the symptoms complex of the patients. At its best, this modification reduces symptoms and at its worse causes side effects, which can increase negative symptoms and even result in death of the patient. Why is this so?

Here is a list of various families of drugs, which give us a clue to the way they function:

- Antihistamines
- Beta blockers
- Serotonin reuptake inhibitors
- Angiotensin blocking agents
- Antibiotics
- COX inhibitors
- Selective estrogen receptor modulators
- Anti-cholinergics
- ACE inhibitors
- HMG-CoA reductase inhibitors
- Leukotriene receptor antagonists
- Proton pump inhibitors

Very clearly what these drugs do is interfere with a physiological function in order to alleviate worrying symptoms in the patient. Any chemical, which can powerfully block a physiological function in order to control that function, could also cause a greater or alternative dysfunction.

In an acute disease this may be very helpful as the body's systems may be losing total control and becoming life threatening. In these cases one does want to calm down the chemical process and powerful drugs can be life saving. Consider the person with a serious life threatening asthma attack, snakebite or massive bee stings. All these people could die following such an attack if it was not for modern medicine.

The drugs are given in high doses for a short period of time. These high doses would not be given in chronic disease where the symptoms are not so acute and life threatening for the simple reason that these high doses for prolonged periods could cause serious harm and even death.

While the drugs are life saving in these situations, one must nevertheless also recognize that underlying all that is happening is the bodies own innate attempt to maintain homeostasis and the body will at some point manage to take over normal function provided the drugs are stopped at some point, allowing this to happen. So while the drugs are life saving they become an interference factor ones the body is back in control and able to maintain balance and harmony.

Healing is a Natural Process Going on all the Time

The above truth cannot be emphasised enough. It is one of the most important and yet least discussed issues in modern conventional medicine. Certainly medical students are taught physiology, which is the study of the normal function of body systems and they know all the different biochemical processes and how normal function is maintained and yet, when it comes to the treatment of disease, it seems that drugs have a priority over the bodies own inherent natural healing processes.

Disease is not a deficiency of drugs and using drugs then is an attempt to control functions in order to alleviate symptoms and does not improve health by supporting the innate healing responses of the body.

Disease is not a deficiency of drugs

In saying that 'disease is not a deficiency of drugs' and therefore why use drugs at all, I am aware that many doctors and the public generally and genuinely believe that somehow drugs are used by medical doctors to treat the disease and therefore heal the person.

If one examines this statement carefully however then it becomes obvious why this idea is actually untrue. What is true is that symptoms can be dramatically improved and even life saving effects can happen with drugs: but does the disease go away and is its progress stopped?

Let's examine a few conditions and discover what is actually going on.

Hay fever and asthma may be treated with antihistamines, cortisone and other 'disease modifying' drugs. All these drugs can alleviate the symptoms. An injection of cortisone can stop hay fever attacks for many months and even for a whole season, asthma is certainly helped and perhaps many people's lives saved by treatment, but is the disease cured and are the risks of side effects over the long term worth the benefits?

In one recent study[1] (2015) published in a peer reviewed journal, anticholinergic drugs use over many years showed a significant increase in dementia and Alzheimer's disease. Anticholinergic drugs include many over the counter drugs to treat hay fever, asthma, insomnia and some bladder problems. These drugs work by blocking acetylcholine, a chemical involved in the transmission of electric impulses between nerve cells and thus the drug shuts down this pathway in a rather haphazard way. Short-term use may not stress the body and helps acute symptoms but long-term use over years is another matter.

Side effects of cortisone in its many forms include bleeding and ulceration when used locally in the nose, cataracts and glaucoma, diabetes, immunosuppression, retardation of growth in children and bone thinning in adults.

Every drug has its list of side effects and the usual story from medical doctors is that the benefits are worth the risk. This may indeed be so when used short term i.e. weeks only but long term use is another matter. Long-term studies are not really available for most drugs and certainly for the kind of combination of drugs now used by so many people.

Millions of people worldwide are taking between three and eight drug combinations. There is no research to indicate how safe this is. The public domain is where the trial is being done. That is to say that anyone taking more than two drugs at a time is taking part in a massive research project. Most drug trials last a few years only and are assessing only one or two drugs at a time.

The long-term use of multiple drugs with powerful physiological effects on the body used by adults for the long haul is not known. People die anyway of a disease and the connection between the drugs taken and the end stage disease may never be known. Drug companies for obvious reasons, are not going to do this research or pay anyone to

1   Gray SL et al Cumulative use of strong anti cholinergic medications and incident Dementia. JAMA .2015; 175(3): 401-407

do it either. The public, they say, is demanding these drugs and to an extent they are right.

Take for example Viagra for women. Women are demanding that such a drug is available for them also. It seems that relatively healthy individuals are prepared to be volunteers for new drugs no matter the consequences. Drugs are known to be the 3rd or 4th most common cause of ill health and death. The public needs to understand that all drugs interfere with function and while the story is that the benefits are worth the risk, this generally only applies to the following:

- The use of a single drug

- When used for the short term

- If the person is relatively healthy, not obese and a non-smoker.

If a person is taking more than one drug over the long term and in addition has a poor lifestyle then there is a good chance that the benefits may not be worth the long-term risk.

Is Prozac more important than the body's own neurotransmitters and does it act in a physiological way? An article in the South African Journal of Psychiatry suggested that drugs are even more natural than natural products as they fit so perfectly onto receptor sites that one would not be amiss in believing that they were tailor made for these sites.

Certainly they are tailor made for these receptor sites by chemical engineers, but doctors may be deluded into thinking that therefore they are working naturally. The authors compared anti-depressant drugs to St. Johns Wort (Hypericum), a natural herbal remedy for the treatment of depression.

Compared to Hypericum, drugs are simple molecules with a very narrow and one pointed focus. In general drugs are developed to block receptor sites and in this way change and even interfere with functions. Hypericum in contrast is a broad, highly complex structure with many active centres. It is so complex that researchers have great difficulty in defining exactly how it produces its anti-depressant effects.

It contains for example the following plant group; flavonoids, phenolic acids, Tannins, napthodianthrones, phloroglucinols, volatile oils, saturated fatty acids, alkanols, vitamins, essential oils and other chemical compounds. While some are actives and other inactives that does not mean that the inactives take no part in the total effectiveness of the plant.

This speaks to our inability to understand the complexity of natural products. Drugs, which are relatively simple, by comparison can be much more easily subjected to a reductionistic science in which a simple chemical is found to block a chemical process in the body.

To conclude that drugs are more natural, because they function in such a simple way and fit perfectly on receptor sites, appears to my mind to be extremely arrogant and have little sympathy for or understanding of the complexity of natural processes. Drugs in the end, despite fitting perfectly onto receptor sites, produce side effects, which may be even life threatening, while natural remedies despite their complexity seldom produce serious side effects. There is good reason for this.

While drugs may fit perfectly on the receptor site and in this way block their function, there is something seriously disturbing about this approach. Firstly it is the assumption that blocking receptor sites and decreasing symptoms in this way is good for the system as a whole and secondly that the power of drugs is what makes them superior to natural products.

Let's have a look at these two assumptions.

Drugs block receptor sites

What happens when drugs block receptor sites? The body's healing systems are always doing the best they can do, even when ill health or even disease are present. In other words even when ill health or disease is present this is nevertheless the best the body can do to maintain harmony and balance.

The human system on one level is into survival and has amazingly robust mechanisms to survive even under seriously disadvantaged positions. Many of the problems of ill health arise from the fact that serious environmental toxins are already blocking and distorting receptor sites. This is aggravated by nutritional deficiencies and imbalances of omega 3 to omega 6 ratio's, which cause dysfunction of the receptors.

When drugs are used to block a receptor site and the body is already doing the best it can to maintain balance, then a reorientation must occur to continue to maintain balance despite the drug's input. The drug has shifted everything in order to alleviate symptoms and the body systems must adjust to this.

The drug itself has no intelligence but the innate intelligence in the body is highly co-ordinated and intelligent. This intelligence must now deal with the fact that the drug has change the name of the game. Other symptoms may now occur and this is called side effects of the drug when in a way this is really the systems of the body shifted to another position in order to maintain balance.

Here is an example of what occurs

SSRIs are 'serotonin reuptake inhibitors'. The assumption is that in people who are depressed serotonin in the brain is deficient i.e. depression is a serotonin deficiency problem. Clever researchers have therefore found ways to prevent the body from removing serotonin and thus increasing the levels in the brain.

The innate intelligence within the system however as indicated before is always doing the best it can do under the circumstances, so that the biochemical background of the person depressed was the best the system could do under the pressure of the causes which as indicated in previous chapters are not simple but complex. When a drug is thrown into the mix the body systems will immediately try and readjust the biochemical profile to return the system to its previous condition i.e. the condition before the drug was given.

This would mean a reduction in the serotonin production because the uptake has been blocked and even a reduction of receptor sites around the body making less available for serotonin action. All this in order to compensate for the fact that serotonin uptake has been blocked and more is therefore accumulating. This accumulation is not what the body required in order to maintain the harmony it had established. While the harmony established may not have been exactly normal, it was nevertheless the best the body could do taking into account all the other factors required to maintain homeostasis.

So while using drugs may help in some cases of depression, it does this by forcing the body intelligence to find another way to maintain the best homeostasis it can under the circumstances. We now know of course that depression does not seem to be a serotonin deficiency problem nevertheless doctors go on using these serotonin blocking agents, forcing the body systems to make a range of adjustments that over the long term will cause increasing stress within the body systems trying to adjust to the drugs interference.

All drugs are powerful enough to interfere with a function. The attitude of most doctors is that they know what the problem is and that it is okay to block that function even though they have no idea how the body as a whole must now balance and maintain a range of functions that are connected.

Blocking cholesterol production is just another example of this management approach. High cholesterol is thought to be associated with increasing heart disease so doctors try to reduce the cholesterol levels using drugs (statins) which block the melevolate pathway (this is the pathway for cholesterol production).

Drug companies normally try and block pathways as close to its end point as possible in order to avoid unintended consequences of blocking too close to the origins of the pathway. All statins however block the melevolate pathway pretty close to its origins. This is the Achilles heel of the pathway and the easiest place to insert a chemical block. Not only does blocking the pathway at this point interfere with cholesterol production but also what is now apparent is that this pathway also produces Co-enzyme Q10, selenium and catechol production.

Well, guess what, Coenzyme Q10 is an essential nutrient for mitochondrial function. The heart cells have the greatest amount of mitochondria of all the cells in the body because the mitochondria produce the energy for heart action. The heart never stops moving and needs lots of the energy produced by the mitochondria. Selenium is essential for immune function and catechol for brain function. Not surprising some of the side effects of statins includes muscle pain (mitochondrial dysfunction), immune disturbances and forgetfulness. Cholesterol is essential for cell membrane and brain health.

Therefore both statins used to bring down cholesterol, a really vital nutrient for a range of functions, and SSRIs which block the uptake of serotonin are both very powerful and serious blocks to important physiological processes. Unintended consequences are inevitable when scientists are dealing with unique chemical profiles of each person and are unable to predict how that drug will impact on that particular individual. To a large extent this is a hit and miss situation and why side effects are so common and why drugs don't always work.

Drugs block biochemical functions and this leads to the side effects.

Natural products

So are natural products 'medicines' and should they therefore be used in the same way as drugs and even regulated within the same framework? Health regulators like to think of any substance packed in a container and sold to the public for health promotion or treatment of disease as a 'medicine', especially if the product makes some kind of claim.

Let's unpack this a little and see what we are talking about.

Drugs and Natural products both treat disease!

Is this true?

This is not entirely true and is in fact a distortion of the truth. Treating and healing are not the same process. Drugs treat and natural products aim to heal. That latter statement is much closer to the truth.

Drugs don't heal. Only the natural healing capacity of the body has the intelligence and capacity to heal. If healing is not happening then there are either blocks in the system (toxins, emotions) or deficiency of nutrients.

Drugs treat by blocking physiological processes

Natural products support healing processes

Natural products are as powerful as drugs.

Natural products as indicated already are not nearly as powerful as drugs. Drugs must be powerful if they want to achieve serious blocking and interference of a physiological function. Most natural products when used in appropriate doses are weak in comparison. They are generally not used for their strength but for their appropriateness to 'support' physiological functions.

There are no effects and side effects of drugs but only effects or side effects. The drug effect is also a side effect.

Natural products on the other hand are not powerful enough generally to block a physiological function. If they were that strong then side effects and even death would be as common as they are with drugs. Side effects even when taken in high doses are extremely rare apart from minor nausea, gastro-intestinal disturbances and occasionally allergic reactions to herbs. Poor quality-controlled herbs may be contaminated by metals but that is another matter.

While the body is not deficient in drugs, it may certainly be deficient in a range of nutrients which can include any one or more of the vitamins, minerals, trace elements, fatty acids, amino acids, simple carbohydrates and other nutrients required for healthy functions.

Many individuals with certain genetic traits require larger amounts of certain nutrients, different calorie requirements, or a particular blend of nutrients and even water.

Do these nutrients become medicines when packed in capsules or tablets and people are given instructions how to take them and how they could improve functions of the body. Is water or food a medicine when given in a particular way for ill people? Have you not seen books written about 'Food as medicine' or the 'waters of life' for healing? Even natural sea salt has medicinal properties.

Do natural products like vitamins and minerals become 'medicines' when they are encapsulated or made into pills and when standard physiological claims are made for them. This is when it gets tricky. Regulators in government want to classify all natural products as 'medicines' and then regulate them like drugs. In some countries there is a separation in regulation between natural products and drugs but this is not the norm. Attempts are generally being made to draw all products, both drugs and natural products, into the same regulatory process causing serious problems for natural products which cannot be patented and therefore get eliminated in the process.

The special case of herbal medicine.

Do herbs treat disease and therefore work like drugs or do they support healing processes?

Herbal products are more problematic because of their complexity; nevertheless they have a history behind them. They were used long before health practitioners knew much about physiology but at a time when the practice of medicine was to support health. Poisonous herbs were seldom used. The conventional paradigm of medicine struggles with herbal medicine because the herbs do not fit into easy categories. They are complex and often even have seemingly opposing chemical families.

Black tea for example has both a stimulant (caffeine) and a sedative (L-theanine) in it. Herbs also have a range of vitamins, minerals, trace elements, hormone like structures, immune boosters and diuretics all in one package. This is very messy to work with and therefore attempts are made to try and reduce this complexity to a more simple active ingredient. Even when this is managed the side effect profile remains exceedingly low compared to drugs like panado and aspirin, popular over the counter (OTC) preparations. When used by trained and experienced herbalists, herbs are exceedingly safe and the vast majority of well known herbs used for hundreds of years by indigenous peoples of that area have never resulted in the amount of deaths caused by common drugs used daily by consumers.

So do herbs treat a condition in a similar way to drugs or do they support healthy functions within the body? There are some toxic herbs, which are seldom used by herbalists for the simple reason that they are toxic and therefore require much care. Most herbs are not used for their toxic effects but because the total combination of their contents are supportive to improving the functionality of body systems.

Herbs support functionality of body systems.

Summary

Drugs are synthetic chemicals, which are very clearly developed to block or interfere with a biochemical process in the body and thus relieve symptoms. They are powerful and dangerous and responsible for thousands of deaths every year nevertheless doctors believe that the benefits are worth the risk. This may be true in the short term provided you don't have a major threatening poison effect but the consequences of long term use in combination generally with other drugs cannot at this time be known for the simple reason that such studies would be too costly and not even feasible.

This means that each person is out there on their own taking a cocktail, which give them symptomatic relief using drugs, which are often given to counteract the side effects of other drugs, and no one really knows how the particular biochemical individuality of each person is going to react or respond to the combination.

Natural products on the other hand are not used for their poison effect but to support physiological functions that are deficient and to maximise functions that are underperforming. It's easy to understand how vitamins, minerals and other similar products used by the body can do this.

In coming back to the questions around regulations for medicines, one must first clearly define two categories of medicines:

- Synthetic chemicals not found in nature and used to interfere with a physiological function.

- Natural products, which are bioidentical to those found in nature and used to support healthy functions.

230

Once there is clarity in this regard then the regulations become fair and appropriate. This is apart from GMP (good manufacturing practices), which everyone agrees are necessary.

There is also the question of efficacy. This is another sticky question that hangs around discussions of natural medicines and is often brought up by its antagonists who regard all natural medicines as just a placebo effect. That accusation seems strange indeed when the amount of nutrient deficiencies present today in large swathes of the population is well known especially in the toxic, synthetic, high sugar refined foods eaten by both the rich and extremely poor. Why would drugs be more useful in the population of deficient individuals? Clearly what they need is nutrient dense foods and even extra nutrients to upregulated systems in the body that require these nutrients to function. These cannot be regarded as placebos.

Are these protagonists then referring to the herbs as placebos. Here again this seems strange indeed when many of the drugs used today have emerged from research on herbs and plants. It is in this kingdom of nature that pharmaceutical companies search for the active ingredients that they can synthesise and modify in a way that makes it possible to patent.

Ah yes, of course it is the homeopathic medicines that really confuse protagonists and this clearly places a smudge on all natural medicines. Homeopathic medicines must be placebos since the manufacturing process includes a technique of diluting the original concentrate until no molecules of the original substance are left and the process includes the strange habit of shaking between dilutions.

I have performed this process many times using the patient's own blood. We used one drop of blood and diluted it in 100 drops of 25% alcohol and kept dilution it over and over again with shaking between each dilution until the 5th, 7th, 9th and 12th dilution. This particular technique was used mainly in children using their own blood to treat their own particular condition. It was my most successful treatment for hay fever, asthma, chronic gastro-intestinal conditions, recurrent colds and poor immune function. I cured children of these conditions when recurrent antibiotics had failed over and over again.

The problem we have here is that there is pretty little left of the original substance, which in the above case was one drop of blood. How can this therefore have any effect on the body and so it must be a placebo effect say the protagonists. This accusation is always strange to a person who has been using the technique for perhaps twenty years, given it to children and even babies where the placebo effect is unlikely and where conventional medicine had already failed.

How to explain the effect of such low power medicine like homeopathy. As Nils Bohr, one of the fathers of quantum science said on receiving the Nobel price for physics: 'I have examined matter all my working life, and I can tell you one thing about matter, there is no such thing as matter, only energy-information.'

So matter is not exactly what we think it is. Matter is energy-information and not surprisingly even information can move energy and matter. So a small pressure on the button of a hand held electronic item can open a heavy gate, which the person would not be able to do with that finger alone. In diluting the one-drop of blood or herbal tincture the 'matter' component gets diluted to an infinitesimal degree but the energy-informational aspects still seem to remain and may become more powerful as they are 'released' from the attraction to matter. I suspect that homeopathic remedies work at this level.

This is not 'matter' doing the work but just information carried within the structure of the diluting liquid. There is very little incentive to do the science, as this would change the face of medicine as we know it so don't expect to have answers soon to this conundrum. In the meantime there will continue to be serious criticism from people who have no experience in the method, have never tried it and for whom the idea just sounds irrational. I am personally convinced that it works having used it in both seriously acute conditions and chronic conditions where no other drug or natural remedy has worked.

I often tell my patients that drugs come out of the mind of man while natural products come out of the mind of God/GreatMystey/Tao what ever you like to call this space. What I mean by this statement is that drugs are constructed with the logical mind using linear thinking based on the information at hand.

Natural products have slowly evolved through an evolutionary process of which we have little understanding. It always amazes me to realise how dependent for example I am on the oxygen produced by the trees and how the carbon dioxide emitted by my lungs is taken up by the trees. Could it be that the trees and my lungs have evolved together?

All living things in nature have evolved together and therefore have links that are not always obvious to the logical thinking mind. In dissecting a herb into its constituent parts, something of that living dynamic quality slips through our fingers and we are left with the bare bones of something which is no longer living in the way it was before. Indigenous people living close to nature always recognised this and would honour the plants in festivals and on their shrines and holy sites. Plants are not just carbohydrates, fats, vitamins, minerals etc. as discovered by scientists in their laboratories but living organisms that seem even to respond to people's energy fields in positive or negative ways.

There are Chefs that are more than just the sum of their parts when it comes to getting a meal together and the same applies to racing horses, artists, magicians, comedians etc. who may just have the edge on others because of unique qualities they have. They are more than the sum of their parts and it is this 'extra' that cannot be weighed and measured that makes all the difference.

Living systems are more than the sum of their parts.

Drugs are the product of a scientific mind attempting to be in control, and exclude the subjective criteria and qualities. Herbs are really nothing like that. They are so complex that they hide within their matter/energy/informational field, qualities that cannot be exactly exposed by the scientific method much to the chagrin of scientists.

Herbalists mix these herbs in diverse ways and quantities, confusing the issues even more. Herbs are not the sum of their parts and this is why most of the knowledge of herbs has emerged over thousands of years from people working with these herbs and not from scientists examining the herbs in the laboratories. The work in laboratories is interesting and not to be denied, yet the real understanding of a herb, what it can do, how it can be combined with other herbs is really happening in the field in actual practice and this is why it takes hundreds of years for herbalists to accumulate sufficient knowledge in the use of these herbs.

Quantity and objectivity is measurable

Quality and subjective components generally gets lost in measurement yet still has an influence on matter.

Chapter 17

Mrs. DB is 53 years old and complains of a pressure feeling around her ears, which can extend into the area around her throat if severe. She has been to an ENT specialist who could find nothing wrong. Could this be stress related, I ask? Yes, she is very quick to answer, after living for 13 years alone she remarried two years ago and the relationship is causing her much stress.

Most patients I see do believe that stress is the main cause or a major contributing cause to many of their symptoms and signs and are merely waiting for their doctor to ask the key question in order to pour out their heart to their practitioner. The practitioner has little time to spend dealing with emotional issues and is thinking of the next patient in the waiting room and therefore avoids such leading questions or may just write out a prescription for a drug to treat anxiety, depression or a sleeping pill .

Dealing with Stress

What are the components of stress and is there a way to deal with a situation that can't always be changed? It is generally assumed that if the situation can't be changed then the stress will continue and one must do one's best and bear the load.

- 'I guess I must just live with the situation.'

- 'There is nothing I can do about the situation so I will have to suffer through it until something changes.'

- 'I was born to suffer.'

- 'Suffering is my Karma.'

The list goes on and on and so does the resentment, anger, depression, anxiety and all the other defensive mechanisms that people use in order to cope and react to the stressful situation. This is not good for ones health. Feeling depressed and negative also means that every cell in the body is going to be surrounded by the chemicals of depression and stress. There is however, in principle, a relatively easy solution to the problem of stress but one must first understand the mechanics of the stressful process.

Have a look at the person sitting across from you. Can you see the person? Where do you live? Cape Town, Amsterdam, in a house, cave, a building? Where is this stressful situation that causes such heartache?

At work, home, with your partner, your boss? There is actually only one answer to all these questions, but let's take them one by one.

1: Can you see the person? Can human beings be seen? Do you know what your wife/child/partner looks like? If they were angry or sad, how would you know? Obviously there would be signs of their emotional state on their face, the look in their eyes and the posture they adopt; but is it the face that is angry or sad. Could I cut open the face and find the angry or sad person there? The face and the body are not the person who is angry or sad, yet reflects the person. It seems that the person is somehow inside and yet not to be found there with the tools at our disposal.

Is the person inside the body?

Can science identify where this person is?

2: Where do you live? Do I really live in a house, cave or building or a town like Cape Town? I can somehow take my body to Cape Town but do I live there? If I don't live "out there" then where do I live? Perhaps the best one can say is that it seems that I live "within" somewhere. I don't wish to go into any philosophical speculation for the moment about where this within is or whether the within is actually a transcendental state and is therefore both within and without. It is so interesting that everyone uses this 'I' word , as if they know what they are talking about and yet there is no objective measurement of this 'I' . The body is an object but the 'I' appears to be subjective.

3: Where is this stressful situation taking place? We can now ask whether it is inside or outside? If the person is "inside" and the body is only reflecting the person, then the stress must also be inside and not outside. The person is not "outside" and therefore cannot know what is actually happening "out there". What actually happens is that information in the form of colour, sound, taste, hearing and touch passes through the various sense organs to the brain and is then interpreted by the mind. Out of this interpretation comes our understanding of 'reality' out there.

In the diagram the circle represents the body within which appears the response of the person to collective information that appears via the sensory apparatus and the interpretation of the mind. The eyes represent all the sensory organs; so information enters via the sensory organs and is interpreted by the mind. Neurotransmitters which are the biochemical equivalent of the thoughts, are then released.

These neurotransmitters then becomes the experience in the body. Our actual experience of the world is therefore dependent not only on the sensory input which itself is limited by the nature of the sense organs but on the interpretation by the mind. The mind in turn is conditioned by its past experience, conditioning, education, points of view, genetics, toxins etc. It is this background which then interprets the information coming in via the sense organs.

Now let's add a so-called stressful situation into the dynamics.

Stressful Situation

The two eyes (sensory organs) look at the situation and from this information received there is then an interpretion by the mind. This interpretation has a background of conditioning, points of views and other preferences which will give a particular slant to the interpretation.

For a pessimist who has a conditioned background of pessimism any difficult situation will generally be seen as a problem and for the optimist the same situation will be seen as an opportunity. The pessimist will have pessimistic thoughts which not only just sit around indulging themselves in more pessimistic thoughts but these thoughts also have a way of effecting physiological responses in the body so that the person begins to 'feel' pessimistic, while the optimist will be expressing optimism.

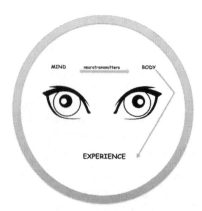

These chemicals are called neurotransmitters. So thoughts are not exactly neutral but will stimulate emotional reactions felt in the body. Even neutral thoughts can influence the body eg thoughts about moving body parts such as lifting the hand. The expression in the eyes, face and body movements will often reveal to another person what is happening within.

Thoughts > move body parts

Can also stimulate emotions felt in the body.

Pessimistic thoughts > pessimistic feelings

Optimistic thoughts > optimistic feelings

Expressed outwardly as body language.

It is in this way that I actually create my own experience which I feel in my body by punching into the computer/brain my description of the situation as it appears to me. If I describe the situation as a problem then my experience become that. If I see the situation as an opportunity then it becomes that for me.

The 'difficult situation' in reality is neither a problem nor an opportunity; it is merely a difficult situation. It becomes a problem in my experience if I call it that and it becomes an opportunity if I call it that. Is a glass with water up to the half way mark, half full or half empty? Well it depends doesn't it. It depends on what you decide to call it. Call a difficult situation a problem and you will experience it as such because the computer brain will obey your orders.

There are also other choices for a difficult situation. How about deciding that God is in that situation. Hello God this is a very difficult situation, but I know you are also present here, I wonder what it is you are trying to teach me, how can I be of service, in what direction are you trying to direct me? So here I am punching God into the computer and my experience will become the experience of the presence of God.

Without realising it we are creating our own reality by the words we use to describe the situation. So if one is stressed then how about looking at the words you are using to describe the situation. The stress is not "out there" because that is not where you are. Sitting inside and looking out the window you are making the decision, which will create the condition you will now experience. So if you don't want to feel the situation as a problem then take some care not to see it as problematic but rather as an opportunity or see the presence of God in the situation or just recognise it as a journey you are on and a bridge over a river that needs to be built in order to get to the other side. What you punch into the computer creates your reality rather than the situation itself.

We create our reality by the words we use to describe the situation.

No one can make you angry or sad or resentful. You create your own reality by the words you punch into the computer. You decide to become angry or sad because of the situation but you could choose another way to look at the situation so that you don't feel so uncomfortable. The extent to which you can change your mind will dictate the level of change you will experience. There are obviously levels of optimism as there are levels of sadness or anger. Those levels are also dictated by conscious and often unconscious decisions that one makes.

'But how can I change my mind if the situation is really a problem?'

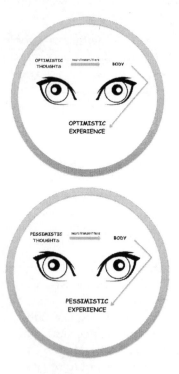

- if my husband is really abusive.

- if I could be without a job.

- if I lost all my money.

- if I had cancer?

If I refer to all these situations as problems, then they are problems to me. The best way to have a problem is to call a difficult situation a problem, but it is important to understand that it is only the mind that makes the choice. So how should I deal with a situation that 'really is a problem'? As indicated, if you call it a problem, then it becomes one for you, but it is not just a question of calling it an opportunity, but of recognising that it is an opportunity and that this requires a little bit of introspection, meditation , contemplation and even quick wittedness. The latter is a useful quality because habitual patterns are extremly powerful and one needs to be very mindful of the games the mind plays.

What is perhaps important is a decision regarding the philosophy one wants to live by. Being an optimist or a pessimist or a believer in a higher Intelligence is a decision that we all need to make. Without such a decision a difficult situation will be decided by our particular mood of that time or what everyone else is saying about the situation.

Choose a philosophy that will help to give you the experience and feelings you would like to live with.

So is it possible to clarify our attitude and philosophy to life so that we can deal with situations more appropriately. Without this clarity, life becomes a choatic expression of our own chaotic mind. We will tend to be optimistic when life is going well and pessimistic when life is not working for us.

This does seem a strange way to live when much better options are available.

So right now decide to become an optimist because it is the one way to begin to feel better about the world and what is happening. It may not be easy to start off with because if you have had a difficult life and suffered from depression much of that life then having someone tell you just to be optimistic does not seem very helpful. But you do need to start somewhere and just recognising how your thoughts can influence how you feel is a good start. Watch how easily a negative thought moves very quickly in creating negative feelings and emotions and that you are doing it to yourself.

No one can climb into your mind and 'press your buttons' of pessimism. You are doing it to yourself because you are the only one inside. Be gentle with yourself and start slowly using positive thoughts even when you feel pessimistic and depressed. Listen to positive talks, listen to music that tends to support positive feelings, watch comedies and use prayer and positive affirmation every morning and evening.

In a recent Time magazine I was reading there was an article on 'The secrets of Super Siblings'. They describe one father who every evening while his three daughters slept whispered into their ears 'I can and I will'. He said that he was talking to their subconscious, 'That's the one that really listens' he said. In the morning, they did a series of jumping jacks, looking in the mirror and said 'Today is going to be a great day. I can and I will'. Even those children who had grown up in a rat infested apartment became respected and successful professionals.

We need to start somewhere and just knowing that it is not the situation that is making you feel the way you feel , that no one can actually press your buttons, but rather it is your thoughts stimulating the neurotransmitters of negative feelings that is responsible for your experience. That is a good start.

Starting to take responsibility and stop blaming others, situations, governments will slowly turn the wheels in the direction you want to go in order to feel the way you want to feel.

Choose to be an optimist even when feeling pessimistic.

Seek out optimistic people, books, music, pray

Even while resting listen to good music or great affirmations.

If you decide to become an optimist then there are still two choices you can make. Either you can decide to be an unconditional optimist or a conditional optimist. A conditional optimist means that it will not take much for that person to become pessimistic again. The person will have a ceiling above which the person again becomes pessimistic.

Choosing to be an unconditional optimist under all circumstances makes much more sense as the chances of feeling good are much more likely than if you are allowing the monkey mind to decide happazardly how you are going to meet the situation. I have been told that optimists are not realists. The real world is full of problems, disasters, misfortunes, tragedies and catastrophes and while some of them may turn out to be opportunities they are in fact all-problematic and cause enormous stress.

All soldiers have to go through obstacle courses in their training. Is the obstacle course a problem or opportunity? Again it depends on the mindset of the person and not on the obstacle course. The obstacle course is there to make a better soldier and not to kill him or her.

My staff will often come into my room with a look of alarm and refer to an opportunity waiting for me outside. Generally I would say to them: 'Okay maybe this is a difficult situation but let us try and turn it into an opportunity by the way we are thinking about it.' It is that process of trying to turn a difficult situation into an opportunity that makes all the difference and starts a process of healing and turns a destructive and unhappy condition or situation into a creative positive one. It may take some effort and will-power to do this and be more or less successful, but nevertheless the principle hold true.

A Positive Attitude will make one Feel much Better within Oneself than a Negative Attitude

Let me give some examples of this process.

A patient is told that she has breast cancer. Problem or opportunity? Well it depends doesn't it, but can cancer be an opportunity? I have seen many men and women where the diagnosis of cancer has been a real wake-up call. Suddenly each moment becomes precious, no time for regrets, time for forgiveness, time to love more, time to savour each moment, time to become as positive and optimistic as one can. A negative viewpoint has been shown to be detrimental to one's health and will support the disease rather than the health. So whose side do you want to be on?

Mr TJ has had ulcerative colitis for 3 years. A lot of hard work and much treatment has at last paid off and he is much better than he was, but in order to get to this point he has had to give up his work and go into early retirement. He still, however, has a great deal of pain and recently this pain has made him feel depressed. 'I feel that I am worthless and can no longer be a useful citizen, always consumed by my ill health and unable to function normally.'

Many people find themselves in this situation, widowers, hemiplegics, severe arthritics, old age, the list could go on an on, and yet we all know some individuals in this category who, despite all odds, manage to find meaning in their lives.

How do they do this? It is surely not easy but in the end what makes the difference is imagination, intent, willpower and faith in oneself, but in the first place it is the ability to look at life creatively and choose the high road.

To do this one must recognise the choices available and see one's apparent handicap as a stepping stone to something different in life to what one had before, to recognize that life is not attempting to cast you aside but rather to shape you for another mission, to give you another direction, to draw your energies for a particular need of spirit. As you allow your imagination to move in this new direction with creative thinking and call up the will to do, then life very often opens up doors in a most unexpected way.

Reality is not made only of hard objects but also soft feelings, emotions, thinking and imagination which are all fluid and flexible.

In my own life I am aware of two main voices, which seem very often to be barking at each other. The one is positive, encouraging, nourishing and supporting while the other is discouraging, confusing, agitating, negative and even destructive. I have decided to no longer listen to the latter voice. What a relief to have finally made this decision and yet it is still surprising how often I find myself in a very mechanical way still listening to this negative voice. When this happens I am now acutely aware of the process, stop feeding into the drama with more negative thoughts of blame or judgment and wait for the healing of time to dissipate the energy of conflict.

Stress management in principle is a simple process of changing ones mind and choosing a story that works. No one out there can make you angry. You choose to become angry because of what the person is doing or saying. It is always your choice. The more happy you are the more happy you will feel, the better the environment you create for cell function and the more happy you will make others feel. Try it.

Chapter 18

He had come to see me for his shoulder problem. The pain had begun about one year ago and he had already been to a physiotherapist and received two cortisone injections from his orthopaedic specialist. The pain had however continued to worry him with very little improvement all this time. I decided to treat him with my low energy laser.

I should explain that the low energy laser is very low powered, causes no sensation and can be used instead of acupuncture needling. One places the laser over the acupuncture point, presses the button, which then switches off after 20 seconds. Then one moves to the next point. The laser light cannot be seen as it is in the infrared range of the spectrum. In some cases immediate results may be seen so that I was not surprised when the patient noted that the pain felt much better after the first treatment.

He was booked to return a few days later. It was only when the next patient came in for laser treatment that I noted that the electrical connection to the laser had been switched off all the time, so that while I had been moving the laser around and the timer had been recording the 20 seconds, the laser light part had not been working and yet the patient had felt much better afterwards.

I expected him to return and complain that nothing had changed. In fact the opposite happened. He was delighted with the treatment and said that this was the first time he had really felt a significant change. He continued to improve over the next few weeks but the biggest shift was that first treatment.

'Any therapeutic meeting between a conscious patient and a doctor has the potential of initiating a placebo effect.[1]'

1   Hrobjartsson A The uncontrollable placebo effect. Eur J Clin Pharmacol 1996.50, 345-348

The Placebo Effect

An enigma that no one wants to look at

The Placebo Effect Defined

The word 'placebo' means in Latin 'I will please' and possibly suggests that the patient is trying to please the practitioner. It is clearly more than just a response to a sugar coated pill but includes a response to the environment, the doctor's attitude, the other personnel in the doctor's office and even just the fact of making an appointment.

Clients will often say that the moment they made an appointment they already started to feel better and I had one patient who told me that if she was ill she would first drive past my place and if she was not better after than she would make an appointment. I should mention that my place is in the country and a half Km along a dirt track so driving past my place is a healing experience in its own right.

'Placebos are getting more effective' and 'drug makers desperate to know why' were recent news headlines. Why would drug makers be at all interested in the 'placebo'? After all, it is seen as just a gimmick pill, without any known chemistry to influence the body, a dummy pill that works not by its chemical structure, but rather by a direct response within the body that it seems has to be mind over matter. Nevertheless the placebo is a most serious problem to drug manufacturers.

From 2001 to 2006 for example the percentage of new drugs withdrawn from Phase 11 clinical trials, when drugs are first tested against placebos rose by 20%. The failure rate in Phase 111 clinical trials increased 11%, mainly due to poor showing against the placebo. This is clearly a serious blow to companies spending millions of dollars on research especially if the placebo response is increasing.

The drug looks great in phase 1 and everyone gets really excited but then suddenly when compared to a sugar coated tablet it really no longer looks exciting and the researchers have to return back to their drawing boards. The result has been that fewer and fewer new drugs are appearing on the market and those that do eventually get through the long process become very expensive, all because of their inability to beat the sugar pill.

Drugs vs. a sugar coated pill. Is it all in the mind?

It seems strange indeed that there should be any controversy around the fact that the mind can influence the body. It is a common experience that the body responds to thoughts and is affected by emotions, and yet the medical profession as a whole seems to have a very ambivalent approach to the placebo response and treats it as a member of the family that they don't like to talk about. One would almost think that using a placebo was unethical, bad medicine and even irresponsible medicine. Now why would a simple pill without any possibility of side effects, and easy to administer, cause such reactions?

Pharmaceutical companies would like to wish the placebo response away, and are generally desperate to undermine and minimize the placebo effect, casting it as the demon in the clinical research programme, as if it spoils their game, and indeed it does. If the placebo response is getting better then pharmaceutical companies will soon be out of business.

A French physician in the 19th century Armand Trousseau is alleged to have said 'you should treat as many patients as possible with new drugs while they still have the power to heal'.

So what is it that pharmaceutical companies don't like about the placebo response, when the placebo effect may be the most important healing stimulus that we know? The truth of course is that the placebo spoils all the fun. It can make the drug look pretty ineffective when so much money was spent to develop the drug.

Drug companies hold their breadth at the end of a drug trial because they know that if the placebo response in that trial is good, then their drug will be shown not to be any more effective than the placebo. Not only is the placebo a confounding factor in drug trials, but in truth one needs to recognize that it is the confounding factor in any form of healing, including faith healing, acupuncture and whenever healing is the result of an interaction between two people, whether a non-pharmacological agent is used or any other symbol or act is used instead.

Could miraculous healing be a 'placebo' response?

Drug trials may not be the best environment for optimum placebo responses either. One would expect that a good placebo response would be more likely if the group of individuals used in the trial were easily affected by the conditions of the trial and if the people were generally optimistic and hopeful of good results. Generally however the conditions of the trial are not supportive to the placebo response, volunteers may be doing it for the monetary gain, doctors are trying to be unbiased and not create any impression that the 'new' drug could really make any difference and generally the environment in which the trial is being done is 'clinical' and not conducive to generating a positive response.

All this is terribly confusing and why drug trials and their results have to be assessed very carefully, and why repeating drug trials may just confuse the issues if the placebo response in one trial is really good but not so good in another trial.

In one study comparing the treatment of peptic ulcers using the same drug in different hospitals (one government hospital and the other a private hospital) the placebo response varied between 25% and 45%. Guess which hospital had the best placebo response. That's right …the private hospital.

So clearly if you want to get a good drug outcome then choose to do your drug trial in a non-privately run health centre and not with people who are interested in the outcome. Paid volunteers and other disinterested individuals may change the placebo response dramatically enough to make the drug look pretty good i.e. the placebo response in these cases is really poor so that the drug appears to work.

In another astonishing trial, surgeons decided to check if the operation they were doing for angina pectoris was really making a difference. Ligation or cutting off of an artery just below the sternum (internal mammary artery) had received wide attention in the 60's. In this study patients were chosen with symptoms of angina and abnormal electrocardiograms.

One group of patients received the standard internal mammary ligation while the second group had a sham operation (a similar incision was made with exposure of the internal mammary artery but no ligation was performed). The choice of each operation was done in a random way. Patient symptomatic improvement was noted in all cases. Following the operation the chest pain disappeared in many cases in both groups, and the use of drugs decreased, exercise tolerance improved. This operation by other surgeons was stopped as a result of this paper[2].

This was not all though. Drug companies soon discovered that even the country in which a trial was conducted made a difference to outcome and it was the placebo effect that seemed to make the difference.

So let's have a look at the history of placebo research.

History of the placebo response.

Henry Beecher in 1955 wrote a paper on the placebo response, which changed the way drugs were being investigated. It seems that Beecher got the idea about the placebo when he was working as an anaesthetist during World War 2. He noted how a nurse working with him used injections of salt water to relieve the pain of wounded soldiers when morphine ran out.

To his amazement, the bogus injection relieved the soldier's agony and prevented the onset of shock. When he returned home he decided to investigate this phenomenon. He collected together dozens of trials and showed that the placebo response is so powerful that many illnesses may respond to the administration of a pill with no active ingredients.

This is true not only of functional problems like indigestion and headaches, but also for more serious diseases like arthritis and cancer. In Beecher's paper the placebo provided satisfactory relief in 35.2% of cases. What was however even more interesting than this mean figure of all the 28 studies he collected was the actual spread of results.

The placebo effectiveness was between 15 and 58% in the different studies. On an individual level, the response of the placebo was even more dramatic in a few cases. What was especially worrying was that the fact that even the drug response could just be a placebo response.

2   Dimond EG et al Comparison of Internal Mammary Artery Ligation and Sham Oper- ation for Angina Pectoris. Am J Cardiology. 1960; April:483-486

Is the drug response just a placebo effect!

Soon after Beecher's report appeared, the thalidomide controversy causing serious birth defects occurred. The public was aghast and Congress very soon amended the Food, Drug and Cosmetic Act, requiring trials to include enhanced safety testing and placebo control groups. This meant that trials needed to be split in two, with one group receiving the active drug and the second group the placebo with neither the doctor nor the patient knowing which was the active drug.

This kind of trial then became the gold standard for research and was called the "double-blind, placebo-controlled, randomised clinical trial". Double blind because both the patient and researcher did not know which was the drug or the placebo,' randomised because the groups were divided in a random way. For a drug to become registered with the regulatory authorities in most countries today, it must do considerably better than the placebo.

In another study Backman and associates reported in 1968 on the treatment of peptic ulcers and several other gastrointestinal conditions, showing a placebo improvement rate of 92%. In other words 92% of people with peptic ulcers responded to a pill with no active ingredients as if it was an active drug.

Moerman collected 32 different papers in which the placebo was compared to the drug Tagamet in the treatment of peptic ulcers and found a mean placebo response of 45%, with a range of 8 to 83%. Again, while the mean of these 32 different studies was 45%, in one study 83% of people responded to a non-active pill as if it was a drug.

That's pretty good going for a pill that costs almost nothing to produce, can be safely used by anyone and even prescribed by a non-professional, is available everywhere and can be used in pill or capsule form and even developed into a syrup, spray or cream.

The Health Industry and the Ethics of the Placebo Response

Of course all this also applies to the health industry. Do the nutrients or homeopathic remedies really work or is it all a placebo response. Antagonists to natural remedies believe that any response is a placebo response. So this is clearly a serious question and can't be easily answered. I would be the first to admit that the health industry has a good story going for it.

They are purveyors of health and that is a really good sell, but do the remedies really work. There are charlatans out there who capitalize on the placebo response and actually do a lot of good work helping people get better by getting the placebo response activated. I call them charlatans only because they are consciously using this tool in an unethical way and there are ethics around the placebo response.

But then any practitioner worth his salt should be 'using' the placebo response not only because it makes good sense but also because everything about the placebo response is about the doctor patient relationship and the environment in which the consultation happens.

Health practitioners understand the importance of the doctor patient relationship and the practitioners getting good results are often the ones spending time to listen, answering all the patients questions and using treatments and medicines that make sense to the ill person. All this also supports the placebo response and therefore adds to the treatment result.

The placebo response is present both with drugs and natural medicines.

Thousands of drug trials, which include a placebo control, have been carried out over the years since they are legally obligatory. Only if the drug does significantly better than the placebo is its use regarded as efficacious, and only then will it be regulated for use by the various control bodies in each country.

So one can imagine the enormous pressure on scientists to make sure that the trial is done well and works in favour of the drug. The placebo is a powerful competitor. If the placebo response is good and over 60%, then the drug is unlikely to be more effective, whereas if the placebo response is weak then the drug response if it is good will look much better.

The enormous variability of the placebo response means that drug trials are always going to be dependent on the placebo and because the drug itself can also have a placebo response it becomes difficult if not impossible to every separate out what remains as a drug effect. Leaving out the placebo arm as indicated still leaves the placebo drug effect and comparing one drug against another will still be confused by the placebo effect.

The colour, shape, and size of the pill may all contribute to the placebo response. The advertising hype makes an enormous difference to the way the drug is perceived by not only the public but even doctors tend to be swayed by what they hear rather than the science. In addition the doctor's attitudes and the particular environment as we have seen contributes to the way people respond to the placebo.

An example of this was the trial carried out by Harden and associates in 1996[3]. This trial was a double blind, randomised trial of acute headache crises in a group of people who had presented themselves to a busy urban emergency department with high expectations that they would receive powerfully effective therapy.

They received either an injection of one of two analgesic drugs (ketorolac or meperidine) or normal saline (inactive). All three treatments produced a very significant difference in pain reduction, with no significant difference between the three treatments. What was confusing about these results was that both these active drugs had previously been shown to be superior to a placebo in a number of other trials.

This is a classic example of the placebo problem. Firstly, its variability under different conditions, and secondly how the placebo response gives definition to the success or non-success of the drug.

If one looks carefully at drug trials there is the observation that drugs do not give absolutely consistent responses, and this is almost certainly due to the placebo effect. In fact it is my impression that everything depends on the placebo response and it is very difficult to identify a true drug effect in most situations. How does one separate the drug effect from a placebo response?

In 1998 Bendetti designed a trial using 33 patients who had the very painful operation of thoracotomy and lobectomy for lung cancer. After the operation the patients all received powerful analgesia at 30-minute intervals to control their pain (up to 6 injections).

3   Harden RN et al The placebo effect in acute headache
     management: ketorolac, mepe- ridine, and saline in
     the emergency department. Headache
     1996;36(6):352-6

The next day when the pain returned they were given saline injections instead and their pain dropped an average of 2,5 points over one hour. In a group not receiving any medication (analgesia or saline) the pain continued to increase over the time of observation. So the placebo group had a marked drop in pain while the non-treatment group experienced pain increase. Bendetti was able to identify what he referred to as placebo sensitives. Other studies have however shown that people who have responded previously to placebos do not always respond again in the same way.

Confusing the issue of the placebo is also the fact that the response is noted in many different conditions, many of them severe with pathological changes such as asthma, diabetes, multiple sclerosis, ulcers and Parkinson's disease. People with mental states such as anxiety, depression and insomnia may also respond to a placebo.

Different outcomes have also been noted when patients are treated by different physicians. One physician[4] was three times more effective than another in alleviating pain using inert (placebo) treatment.

The placebo effect is even present in surgery. Dr Bruce Moseley[5], an orthopaedic surgeon with much experience in knee surgery and its very positive results in his hands decided to test which part of the operation gave the patient most relief. The patients in the study were divided into 3 groups. One group had the damaged cartilage in the knee shaved, while the other group had what is typical described as a washout with loose material removed. The last group was the control group and had 'fake' surgery.

The patients were sedated and three standard incisions were made and everyone acted and did what would otherwise look like normal surgery. The results were shocking to everyone concerned. Said Dr Moseley: 'My skill as a surgeon had no benefit on these patients. The entire benefit of surgery for osteoarthritis of the knee was the placebo

4   Sarles H, Camatte R et al A study of the variations on
      the response regarding duo- denal ulcer when treated
      with placebo by different investigators. Digestion
      1977; 16: 289-92
5   Moseley JB et al A controlled trial of arthro- scopic
      surgery for osteoarthritis of the knee. NEJM. 2002;
      347(2):81-88

effect'. People in the placebo group were even able to play basketball and walk in a way they could not do before the surgery.

Not only can the placebo heal a person of his or her ailment, but also astonishingly it may even have side effects, especially if the side effects of the drug that the placebo has replaced are known to the patient.

Side effects from the placebo! The Nocebo response

The Nocebo response is opposite to the placebo response, but shows again the confusing state of research when human beings are concerned. In this response taking a placebo is associated with negative effects. This is not uncommon in any drug trial where a placebo is also given.

Nausea, dizziness and headaches are common "side effects" of the placebo. Clearly if people are responding to expectations, and if they believe that they are taking a powerful drug, which has side effects, then, side effect to the placebo may happen. When normal coffee is replaced by decaffeinated coffee in a double-blind crossover study (the coffee drinkers don't know that the switch has taken place) they still react by developing a tremor after both drinks, and in another similar study testing drunkenness, 27-29% of the subjects were intoxicated by flavoured water when they thought they were drinking alcohol.

What does this all mean?

By now most readers should be asking the obvious questions. If people are responding in such dramatic ways to a non-pharmacological substance, then is it possible that a great deal of the 'drug effects' are also a placebo response, that the expectation of results from drugs is enough to produce results. So while doctors make a big fuss about the positive results of the drug, these positive results may actually be due to a placebo effect and not the drug itself. It is clear why no one wants to even suggest this possibility. Here is a list of some of those reasons:

- The placebo as a pill, capsule or any other form is dirt-cheap and won't make much money for anyone.

- Imagine a pharmacy that sells only placebo tablets for any condition you could want in any form you desire, in any colour that appeals to you and it could even come with a prayer, poem or mantra depending on your believe system. No doctor required, just your belief system in place. Nevertheless research suggests that even if you don't believe in the placebo effect it can still work. I will discuss this later.

• The pharmaceutical industry could collapse if people stopped using drugs.

• People could become empowered to treat themselves.

Surprisingly, doctors actually do use the placebo response in many different ways, and they may not like to admit to this. Many prescriptions that doctors give are just meant to be a placebo in their minds, and to pacify the patient's need for a pill that they believe will deal with their symptoms.

If both placebo and nocebo effects are real, then why is research not being directed towards identifying ways to facilitate healing with non-invasive, body-friendly approaches to healing. Are drugs really necessary? We come here to the crux of a deep-seated problem which also gives insight into the way business works. Medicine is as much about making money as it is about dedication to helping people. Depending on who is involved, the pendulum may be more on the side of making money or on the side of helping people to recover from ill health.

Do we need drugs if the placebo works so well?

We do know a lot already about the placebo response.

1. The most important factor about the placebo response is the patient's expectation. It seems that the slightest trace of expectation can influence the results of the treatment. When the patient has an intravenous drip inserted for a period of time, and during that time the drug given for pain is stopped and a non-active substance is replaced unbeknown to the person, then the person will continue to believe that they are still under pain management and not feel any pain.

2. Expectation can be enhanced by a number of acts, conditions and influences:

• The doctor's attitude. A hand on the patient's shoulder, a warm handshake and kind words can make all the difference

• The doctor's waiting room can add to or decrease the level of expectation. People attending private hospitals where the conditions are friendlier respond to placebos generally more often than people attending government hospitals.

• Even the colour, size, form (pill, capsule, powder etc.) of medication and name can make a difference to outcome.

• People in different countries respond differently to a placebo. Prozac for example performed better in the United States than in Western Europe and South Africa. This is very unsettling for drug companies who must decide where to run their trials. It may be the reason why some drug trials are conducted in many countries at the same time in order to dilute this effect.

• The more people talk about the benefits of the drug, the better the placebo response. This may be the reason that over time the placebo response actually gets better so that repeat drug trials on the same drug that had previously given a better result than the placebo may now no longer give better results. Good advertising by the drug companies has increased the expectation of benefit and at the same time improved the placebo aspect of the drug in the public domain and also its associated placebo effect in research trials, confounding the overall results. Drug companies who sponsor these drug trials don't like to repeat a drug trial in which the drug has come out better than the placebo for this very reason. What they do is rather repeat the trial, but compare the drug to another drug rather than a placebo.

• Not surprisingly, even waiting for the appointment or surgery can trigger a healing response which is why so often people arriving at the doctor's office or for surgery no longer have the symptoms they initially complained of. Waiting creates expectation, and this initiates a placebo effect of healing.

Mechanism of placebo response

Three major mechanisms have been proposed to explain the placebo-evoked improvement: release of endorphins in response to the placebo stimulus, the conditioning model (learned response), the meaning or expectancy model. Probably all three models have a place but the underlying factor in each case may be different and even shift as time goes on.

This is clearly a most fascinating area of healing response (placebo effects) and even points to the way that people can make themselves sick (nocebo effects) without any other factor/s involved. In the real world there is no single cause of ill health and the nocebo effect also has other names e.g. mind-body stress effects, psychological factors, psycho- spiritual factors. In addition there are all the other underlying causative factors mentioned in previous chapters such as poor food choices, toxins, lack of exercise etc.

While it is clear that the 'mind' must be involved in the placebo and nocebo effects, it is also not so straightforward. People respond even when they don't believe in the placebo, difficult to remove so-called sensitive's from trials, respond even when told that the medication is only a placebo.

Just as in real life, we all have a range of expectations, wishes and deep desires that don't always manifest or manifest when we least expect. This suggests that the more superficial mind that I refer to as the 'thinking mind' is not really in charge of this process. As discussed in the chapter on 'where are the controls', a deeper part of the mind is in charge. This part of the mind I call the 'knowing mind'. When that part of the mind is triggered then the placebo or nocebo response can be initiated.

Summary

The placebo was initially included into the drug trial process because it was assumed that it was merely a benign substance without any activity. This was clearly a huge mistake and while it still is a substance with no known direct physiological effects, as a symbol of healing it is extremely powerful in the responses it can initiate in the body. Today we also know that the placebo is a package that is much more that the 'pill' but includes the doctor, the environment and the patient.

Individuals can respond in a positive or negative way to symbols and rituals. The symbol may be a pill or tablet, and includes the ritual taking place in the doctor's office but starts even when the patient makes an appointment. From that moment something is initiated in the person's mind/brain, which starts a healing response.

A great deal of what is thought to be the drug effect is just the person's expectation of a result. In one study it was found that 75% of the effect attributed to the perceived use of anti-depressants was actually due to the placebo. The perception of clinical benefit from the anti-depressants seems to be largely due to the perceptions of the mind the patient, and not to the actual chemical make-up of the pills patients were taking[6].

If the 'knowing mind' is so powerful that it can initiate healing more profoundly than the drug, then perhaps it is time to re-assess what we are doing in medicine and find more effective ways to activate the body's own innate healing potential which is what the placebo must be doing.

The work of other research scientists[7] shows that this placebo response is also different to a drug effect and activates different parts of the brain. Drugs work by interfering with physiological processes and blocking or dampening down physiological events. The placebo however works in a very different way, which may have more powerful and far-reaching effects as it operates through the most natural pathways towards healing rather than just treating a symptom.

The placebo stimulates the body's most natural healing responses.

So we are left with a whole range of contradictions and absurdities. The placebo is perhaps the best medicine we have, and the cheapest, yet its use is regarded as unethical, and the medical profession feels very uncomfortable with too much talk about the placebo. It is very difficult to predict who will respond to a placebo, and being nice to a person on a drug trial could spoil the trial for the drug company and waste all the money spent on the trial. While medical doctors like to suggest that homeopathic remedies are just placebos, the same may be said for drugs, and of course the same could be said for any remedy including vitamins and minerals.

Quantum science has the same thing to say about the quantum world. It states clearly that a scientist can't know everything at the same time. If you measure the particle property of light then you can't measure the wave properties and vice versa.

6   Kirsch I et al Listening to Prozac but hearing placebo:
     A meta-analysis of antidepressant medication.
     Prevention & treatment, Volume 1,June 1998
7   Leuchter AF et al Changes in brain function of
     depressed during treatment with placebo. American
     Journal of Psychiatry.2002;159: 122-129

Quantum science also points remarkably to the fact that the mere act of observation changes what is being observed. So the whole process of healing and what initiates healing remains murky. This pleases me a great deal and reminds me to not disregard my own intuitive nudges and to rather find ways to include these inner voices together with the facts of science. These facts I now know are never absolute either but sit on the same shifting sands as my own intuition.

Despite all the amazing potentials of the placebo, one nevertheless needs to keep in mind the complexity and even ethics of what we are dealing with. There are many Charlatans in medicine that understand the nature of mind and take advantage of that. They are also referred to as snake oil salesmen. These people do a lot of good work and a lot of bad work but their ethics are all wrong.

The point is not that placebos work just as well as drugs and perhaps even better in some cases so that drugs are not really necessary. What I am pointing to in this chapter is that healing is a much bigger story than just giving a placebo or a drug or even surgery. Healing is a profound and deeply complex process in which mind in its full and complex form participates towards a healing response.

People who play 'placebo games' with ill patients are unethical in practice because they do not acknowledge the greater reality, even the sacredness of the healing response. The 'greater mind' is far grander than our little thinking egocentric mind and there is more intelligence at work than may seem obvious. As healers we need to respect this process.

May the Great Mystery remain a great mystery. The placebo response is a continual reminder of the amazing testament to the power of the mind-body interaction.

Chapter 19

Her mother had died recently at a relatively young age of porphyria, a genetic trait prevalent is some families. She had been warned that it could reduce her lifespan as well and that she should avoid any sun exposure, which was the precipitating factor for the ill health.

Her question to me was whether something could be done despite the genetics, to support health. That's a good question I said. Is genetics the final arbiter of how long a person will live their lifespan? Which is more important, her genetic background or her lifestyle? This is clearly an important question to answer for this young woman. If it is all in the genes then she might just as well become a fatalist and hope for the best but if environmental factors make a difference then there is a handle in her health-disease status that she needs to be aware of.

Lifestyle Management

Defining the Genome (genetic profile) of human beings promised to confer absolute insight into health and disease. Of course this has not happened for the simple reason that it is now obvious that environmental factors have a great deal to do with the way the genes express themselves. The genes do contain the potential but the environment can enhance, block or direct the potential in many different directions. This is not difficult to understand.

The environment we are referring too actually has two faces. There is firstly the outer environment of the body and secondly the inner environment of the cells and the structures within the cells. Both environments do connect with each other but there is nevertheless very strong filters preventing noxious elements from entering inside the body spaces.

The genes do define what is possible for each species and even set criteria and limits around the use of nutrients and the way these nutrients are processed. Toxins and chemicals in the environment will effect each individual in different ways and to some extent this depends on the genetic makeup.

No gene is an island however. The gene is sitting within a nucleus, which is within a cell surrounded by a cell membrane with another outer environment that surrounds each cell. That extracellular space is alive with activity defending the cells, feeding the cells with nutrients and hundreds of other activities to maintain harmony and healthy functions.

Then there is the world outside the body, which has its own levels of noxious substances and stress factors. The genes are clearly a small part of this whole system requiring their own nutrients, energy supply and support teams in order to function optimally.

One can see from the above that there are many areas in which genes can be influenced both positively or negatively. This constitutes the environment and how it is possible to influence genetic outcomes and why the young woman described above can still make a huge difference to outcome if she understands lifestyle factors and how to optimize health.

There are a number of well-recognised lifestyle factors, which contribute to ill health:

- Poor Food choices

- Being overweight

- Lack of Exercise

- Nutritional insufficiencies

- Toxins in the environment (see chapter 10)

- Drugs (see chapter 16)

- Electromagnetic pollution

- Poor sleep patterns

- Emotional-mental stress

- Psychospiritual factors

Each one of the above factors contributes to ill health and it is probably true to say that in each person with ill health many of the above factors are present to a greater or lesser degree. Toxins are present everywhere, in the water we drink, in the air we breathe, in the food we eat, in toothpaste, cosmetic creams, cleaning solutions, buildings, mattresses etc.

Many toxic chemicals are carried by wind and are present in swimming pools and in the sea, polluting the fish we eat. The drugs people take in increasing amounts are also chemicals, which disturb function, and can give rise to iatrogenic disease (doctor induced ill health and even death), regarded as the 3rd most common cause of ill health.

The burden of electromagnetic pollution is still being debated, but it is highly unlikely that the sensitive human biological system is not affected by the constant and continuous bombardment of electromagnetic waves from cell phones, computers, TVs and other electronic devices around the house, in our work situation and in the environment all around. All this just adds to the increasing dysfunctional load on the body systems

To this load is added the chemicals of emotional stress and auto-toxins (produced in the body via chemical processes) produced in the liver and other parts of the body by the organs and tissues as they become more dysfunctional because of the increasing load of toxins, which cannot be removed sufficiently fast enough.

There are three phases moving from health to ill health and finally disease. Phase One is poor lifestyle, which leads to Phase Two, increasing dysfunction and then Phase 3, the disease.

Phase 1 Poor lifestyle
Phase 2 Increasing dysfunction
Phase 3 The disease

This chapter is all about lifestyle and the choices we make which may be the most important contributor to ill health. Changing lifestyle can do more good to our health-ill health status than any other modality. The food you take out of the department store can be a pretty good indicator of your health status and interest in maintaining health.

Food choices

Why are there conflicting views when all food groups are important? It is sometimes said that there are essential fatty acids and essential amino acids, but no essential carbs and that one could live without carbs in the diet. There is no known dietary deficiency of carbohydrates.

More recent evidence suggests that too stringent low carb diets can have an effect, for example on mucous production leading to constipation, deficient mucous in stomach and the intestine. Mucus carries with it a range of immune protective chemicals. The low carbohydrate diet is often deficient in fibre and many other essential nutrients.

While glucose is regarded as an easy source of energy for the body and brain, there is an alternative source of energy when this is not available, derived from fat and called ketones. The brain can easily use this source of energy. During any form of starvation, fat is broken down into ketones, which can be used as energy.

This means that when there is serious calorie restriction or a low carbohydrate high fat diet, ketones derived from fat becomes the primary source of energy and this is why the high fat low carbohydrate diet will lead to loss of weight and fat provided that an excess of food is not consumed. Generally on a high fat diet, appetite is also diminished.

There is a limited capacity to store carbs as glycogen in the liver, and excess carbs are converted by insulin into fat. Excess carbohydrates are generally the most obvious reason for the increasing epidemic of obesity worldwide. Insulin is a storage hormone to help us deal with famines and days without food by storing carbohydrates as fat, and is not meant to deal with massive amounts of excess calories as carbohydrates that people all around the world, both rich and poor, are consuming today.

It is difficult to compare Paleolithic men and women to modern day humans. A great deal depended on what was available locally, the seasons of the year and the skills of hunting, fishing and fire making. There were times of plenty of food and times of famine so that the human being had to adapt to a variety of foods and different amounts of food available.

Some of the early people ate mainly fat, meat and dairy while on the other extreme people ate mainly root crops, fruit in season, herbs and other vegetation with occasional fish and meat when available. The body can fairly easily switching from glucose for energy to ketones derived from fat.

Many experts today believe that humans still have the genetic makeup of 'hunter-gatherers' who ate a diet of wild animals and vegetation, and that our bodies do not have the genetic make-up to consistently process a high carb diet, especially refined carbohydrates.

Clearly the food available today and the choices people have, is very different to thousands of years ago and even 100 years ago. The the speed with which the diet of people around the world has undergone changes is remarkable. These changes in particular have been towards highly processed foods, which store well without degradation and can be easily transported around the world for sale to people everywhere. This is part of the globalization process.

The driving force for all this has not really been human health promotion but monetary gain. In general, human beings have lost touch with nature and what is good and healthy, for quantity of output and profit margins. Industry and commerce has perfected ways to sell items that are 'clearly' not healthy and even mass-produced foods that no longer have the health vitality of foods eaten by our ancestors. Appearance of fresh products is now more important than the quality.

The astonishing increase of diabetes in China tells us the entire story that is spreading fast throughout the world and why the solution is actually obvious. In China the rate of diabetes were almost zero 25 years ago; by 2007 there were 24 million diabetics and by 2010 there were 93 million diabetics and 148 million pre-diabetics. In the Middle East, nearly 20-25% of the population is diabetic. We are also starting to see young children with type 2 diabetes and adult complications of Metabolic Syndrome.

Americans consume an average of 600 cans of carbonated drinks per year each (50 cans per month just less than 2 cans per day). South Africans consumed 254 cans of Coke per person in 2010, compared with a worldwide average of 89.

Each can (375ml) and depending on the make has an average of 9-10 tsp. sugar and 150 calories, together with 30-55mg caffeine, plus phosphoric acid, which interferes with the body's ability to use calcium and will also, neutralize HCl in the stomach. It is not difficult to understand why obesity is such a major problem today.

Sugar addiction: increasing sugar consumption with high insulin production in sensitive children can lead to a hypoglycaemic reaction causing increasing adrenalin and hyperactivity symptoms followed by a drop in glucose that is then alleviated by consuming more sugar. This causes hormonal mayhem and neurological agitation in children and even many adults. Very important to add more fat and protein and reduce refined carbohydrates.

Diabetes is now epidemic throughout the world with a massive amount of people falling into the prediabetic range. The cause of this massive increase in diabetes over such a relatively short period of time is consistent with the very rapid change in food habits, rather than genetic factors, in particular the increasing amounts of hidden sugar in processed foods available everywhere.

Two food groups have dominated the change and these are refined and processed oils and refined and processed carbohydrates.

The evil pair destroying the health of children and adults:

Refined and processed oils
Refined and processed carbohydrates

Our Paleolithic ancestors ate 22 teaspoons of sugar per year.

At the beginning of the 1800s, the average person consumed 4.5kg a year. Today, the average American eats 68 to 82kg per year. A 600ml sweetened carbonated drink or sports drink contains an average of 17 teaspoons of sugar.

600ml carbonated drink = 16-17 teaspoons sugar

350ml fruit juice = 10 teaspoons sugar

750 ml sports drink = 15 teaspoons sugar

350 ml energy drink = 9 teaspoons sugar

Excess sugar keeps driving up insulin, leading over time to fat storage, insulin resistance and eventually after many years to diabetes type 2. Prediabetes is the high insulin stage before pancreatic islet cells become exhausted.

When this happens and the insulin falls then blood glucose rises and this is the onset of diabetes type 2. The prediabetic phase with the high insulin levels is also called Metabolic Syndrome and during this phase heart attacks are more common. Sugar is not a health food and when taken in excess causes the insulin levels to be constantly stimulated and high in the blood. Diabetes itself is a high-risk disease and causes the person to age almost 10 years earlier than most.

Processed oils are the other group of really poor quality foods eaten in considerably greater amounts than consumed by our ancestors. Oils were always cold pressed with the goodness extracted and used locally before the oils had a chance to oxidize and deteriorate. In todays world, oils are refined to keep stability, prevent oxidation, remove odours and tastes and create an oil that can withstand time, travel, heat of cooking and is neutral in every way.

In order to do this the oils are subjected to a range of processes, which include the use of chemical solvents, steaming at high temperatures, de-waxing, bleaching and deodorising. Many of the chemicals used are even toxins such as hexane which is a neurotoxin and a byproduct of petrol production and a serious toxic air pollutant. Hexane residues may remain in the oil. Many of the fatty acids in the oil are changed into trans fats which themselves may be toxic as well. The de-odorising process is essential to remove the odour of all the chemicals involved in the processing.

There are a number of serious problems arising from refining oils, which like sugar above have also contributed to a serious imbalance in the metabolic processes in the body apart from their inherent toxicity. The imbalance in metabolism arises from a major shift in the natural ratio of fatty acids required in the body to maintain a healthy balance. The generally accepted ratio between the omega 3 and omega 6 fatty acids has generally been 1:1 or 1:2. This has shifted dramatically over the last 100 years to almost 1:20 with people consuming an excess of omega 6 in the processed oils.

In the early part of the 1900 there was no refined oils, so again we need to recognize the role of a major food group in the increase of chronic ill health. One of the major causes of ill health is the increasing inflammation within the body. Guess what, omega 6 fatty acids tend to increase inflammation in the body while the omega 3 fatty acids are anti-inflammatory. Processing changes the structure of these natural molecules and there is no way of knowing the long-term consequences of these denatured fatty acids.

The increasing burden of chronic disease however should direct us away from using items of food that are not only seriously processed, but also taken daily in some form or another and have the potential of causing serious metabolic derangement in the body. There is really no point in waiting for the results of clinical trials.

There is sufficient evidence to stop the use of refined oils and processed carbohydrates immediately and return to eating the most natural foods like butter and even lard and tallow together with cold pressed olive oil and cold pressed coconut oil which has not been processed further to remove its taste.

Essential to understand is the way the body uses fatty acids to build and strengthen cell membranes, brain and nerve health in very definite ratios. The highly processed oils containing oxidised omega 6 oils, which distort the ratio of omega 6 to 3 and cause cell membranes everywhere to be leaky and dysfunctional.

Apart from refined oils and refined carbohydrates the next group of bad food choices must be 'junk foods' or foods that are processed with added chemicals such as preservatives, colouring matter and a range of other chemicals to bleach, soften, enhance the taste using MSG and other synthetic chemicals etc.

Once again we are dealing with food that was almost unknown 100 years ago and that has increased dramatically since then. In flying from one city in china to another city in China I was handed a box, which contained my lunch. Inside the box were about 8 packages. Each package contained dehydrated and processed foods that were unrecognizable to my western eyes anyway. Difficult to believe sometimes how much our food choices have changed within a very short period of time.

Bad food choices:

Refined oils
Refined carbohydrates
Junk foods

Unfortunately that is not the end of the story. A whole range of foods that were once regarded as healthy is slipping very rapidly into the unhealthy category. Stables like meat, fish, fruit and even vegetables now have become suspect.

Animals no longer range freely eating fresh uncontaminated grasses, instead they are often kept in enclosed spaces and prevented from walking around freely, given abnormal feed in the form of grains, much which is GMO derived and other fillers to fatten them quickly, injected with growth hormones and antibiotics.

The story with fish is similar. Farmed fish, which now accounts for almost 40% of the fish sold and eaten today is becoming increasingly suspect as a health food. Farmed fish live in extremely unnatural conditions, crowded together without much space to swim around, fed unnatural foods including grains and sometimes given antifungal and other chemicals to control infestations.

Food choices should be a priority if you are interested in health promotion. Taking drugs rather than removing junk food and refined food from your table makes no sense. Drugs, junk and refined foods only add to the body burden over the long term and will continue to be responsible for the increasing incidence of chronic disease.

Exercise

Exercise may be the most important lifestyle activity to promote health and wellbeing, and this may be even more so as we get older. Exercise will prevent the development of fragility and the increasing fracture risk in older persons. The better and more mobile an older person is, the better they feel and the less dependent on others they will be. Numerous studies have shown that improving levels of physical fitness will delay death and extend life. Fifty to seventy percent reductions in the incidence of heart disease and diabetes can be achieved by diet and lifestyle alone[1]. No drug or even natural medicine can reach this kind of positive benefit.

Exercise has been shown to increase life span by an average of one to four years for people engaging in moderate to difficult exercise routines and those extra years will include better general health with less cardiovascular problem and better muscle tone.

Nor does the exercise need to be vigorous. Just walking briskly for only three hours per week can reduce ones chances of developing many chronic health problems.[2] [3]

Exercise[4] may also alleviate depression as well as enhance self-image and quality of life. Exercise has been shown to improve the quality of life in a range of different diseases including diabetes, stroke,

1   Stampfer MJ et al Primary prevention of coro- nary disease in women through diet and lifestyle. NEJM; 343: july 2000

2   Jonker JT, De Laet C, et al. Physical activity and life expectancy with and without dia- betes: Life table analysis of the Framingham Heart Study. Diabetes Care. 2006 Jan;29(1): 38–43

3   Chakravarthy MV, Joyner MJ, et al. An obligation for primary care physicians to prescribe physical activity to sedentary patients to reduce the risk of chronic health conditions. Mayo Proc. 2002 Feb;77(2):109–13.

4   Rochester CL. Exercise training in chronic obstructive pulmonary disease. J Rehabil Res Dev. 2003 Sep-Oct;40(5 Suppl 2):59–80.

multiple sclerosis, chronic obstructive lung disease and many other conditions.[5]

Routine exercise contributes to thicker and stronger bones and contributes to a much lower incidence of fractures in older people. There is some evidence also that exercise can improve the symptoms of older people with arthritis.

Weight reduction

Obesity and overweight have now become epidemic with some 66% of women and 33% of men in South Africa overweight, and between 10% of men and 28% of women classified as morbidly obese. (Dr Tessa van der Merwe from the Centre of Metabolic Medicine & Surgery).

Of special concern is the number of children now overweight. Up to 5% of boys and a staggering 25% of girls in South Africa are obese or overweight. Only the UK, Canada, the USA and Mexico exceed our poor statistics.

Obesity is weighted the same in terms of ill health as excessive drinking and smoking and is even expected to replace smoking as the most powerful preventable risk factor. It is associated with increased risk of coronary heart disease, arthritis, diabetes, hypertension, dyslipidemia and even some cancers. Statistics suggest that obese people are generally in denial and even regard themselves as healthy provided there are no symptoms of ill health. Unfortunately this is not at all true. Obesity is an illness and suggests that the system is already under stress and out of balance.

The good news is that any weight reduction can result in significant health benefits.

- Australian report 2001: 40% of Australians overweight and 20% obese. Diabetes is precipitated by weight gain and as a consequence 1 in 4 Australians aged 25 or older has diabetes or is at high risk of developing the disease in the next 5-10 years.

5 Church TS, Cheng YJ, et al. Exercise capacity and body composition as predictors of mortality among men with diabetes. Diabetes Care. 2004;27:83–8

- In African American women more than half of those 40 years and older were found to be obese, and 80% overweight.

- The two most influential factors regarding overweight and obesity are food intake and physical activity.

- Before 1940 in most developed countries the food intake consisted of a high intake of cereal products, relatively low consumption of fat and sugar and a high consumption of vegetables and to a lesser extent of fruit.

- This has changed and nowadays the consumption of bread and other cereals and vegetables is much lower, but fat consumption and refined sugar is much higher.

- Physical activity has also fallen dramatically and this is especially a concern among children who spend many hours in front of the TV.

- Smoking, obesity and lack of exercise all contribute to poor health over time. Add stress to the mix and life expectancy will be markedly affected.

What is obesity?

This is defined as 20% above ideal body weight. Muscular athletes however may be more than this, yet be quite lean. A better definition therefore may be defined as a body fat percentage greater than 30% in women and greater than 25% in men.

Waist circumference, which is a measure of central fat distribution, can also be used to estimate health risks related to excess body fat. Measuring at the level of the uppermost point of the iliac crest should not exceed 89cm in women and 101,5cm in men.

What causes obesity?

It used to be thought that when energy intake exceeds energy expenditure, weight increase would occur. Research is now showing that it may be much more complex than this.

Insulin is the hormone that stores the energy as fat. Sugar is toxic in high concentrations so that insulin changes the sugar into glycogen and then into fat. Simple refined carbohydrates stimulate insulin release and storage as fat if not consumed immediately in exercise. High daily consumption of refined carbohydrates (sugars and refined cereals) may condition the body to stay in storage mode.

So here we go again…Storage mode activity, plus no or little exercise, plus chronic stress that increases the bodies cortisol (steroids) levels, plus high sugar (not fat) foods leads to obesity. Having a genetic/familial component does not help either.

- Little Exercise
- High Refined Carbohydrates
- Chronic Stress
- Increased Cortisol
- Increased Insulin
- Fat Producing Inflammatory Cytokines and Hormones
- Low progesterone and Relatively High Estrogen
- Thyroid Malfunction Slowing Metabolism = Obesity
- A Family History of Overweight Individuals

While I personally prefer the Mediterranean style diet for long term health maintenance, the high fat, medium protein and low carbohydrate diet (Banting diet) is generally the fastest way to loose body fat and switch off the high insulin levels causing fat storage.

Sleep

Chronic sleep deprivation has been tied to an increased risk of type 2 diabetes, cardiovascular disease, obesity, and depression.

Sleep research on healthy, non-obese subjects demonstrated a 40% decrease in insulin sensitivity for 'short sleepers' (5 hours/night) vs. 'normal sleepers' (8 hours/night). This means that poor and inadequate sleep will contribute to Insulin resistance, which is a forerunner to the development of Diabetes 2.

Leptin, the hormone of starvation decreases when a person does not sleep well. Person then wakes up feeling hungry and less satisfied after eating. Ghrelin on the other hand rises with poor sleep patterns and increases appetite making it even more difficult to control weight.

The stress of not sleeping also leads to chronic cortisol increases, aggravating weight gains and causing sweet cravings. Insulin is a storage hormone converting glucose into fat so that one can understand that not getting enough sleep may contribute to obesity.

In addition to all these biochemical disturbances is the increasing amount of inflammation due to the hormone imbalance and obesity.

Sleep apnea is a sleep disorder characterised by pauses in breathing or periods of shallow breathing during sleep. This occurs particularly in obese men.

Signs of sleep apnea: awakening regularly with a headache, a dry mouth, and/or in a pool of drool, being told that you snore loudly while sleeping. Sleep apnea affects hormonal balance and often causes weight problems with difficulty in losing weight. There is a strong relationship between sleep apnea and low testosterone levels especially in men but also women.

Most people need at least 8 hours of good sleep for optimum health. I encourage healthy sleep habits which include keeping the lights more dim from one hour before sleep, not watching TV or using computers or other bright lights before bed, not activating sympathetic tone by arguing with partners, friends or even yourself and keeping the bedroom as dark as possible during the night.

Choose natural sleep aids over drugs, which do not provide normal sleep patterns. These include listening to music, a hot bath, massage, herbal teas and reading before bed. A good night's sleep should be regarded as anti-aging, health promoting and rejuvenating. Keep in mind that during the day we become more and more exhausted and that at night the body recharges itself for the next day. It seems that 6 hours is just not enough time for this re-charging to happen.

Stress and Psycho-spiritual factors

I have placed these together so as to clarify what I mean and why they are different.

Stress as I explain it has much more to do with emotional-mental factors while psychospiritual has to do with meaning, journey work, relationship to God or some higher power. Of course nothing in human life is quite that straight forward. Every emotion is mixed up with meaning, feeling and has a background of belief and a particular philosophy that guides ones attitudes and colours ones emotional-mental responses.

Nevertheless one can sometimes pull the weave slightly apart and see the play that is going on within each person. Not everyone wants to go too deep into the psyche and prefers to deal with the more superficial aspects of ego. It is enough for most patients just to have to deal with their emotional-mental life and they don't particularly want to discuss meaning and feelings that arise.

In my personal life every physical symptom I have, every acute infection even such simple conditions such as a cold, 'flu, injury, headache, indigestion are all calls to a deeper understanding of self. They come into my life with a particular purpose or message and are never haphazard. That is my story of course and I don't necessarily impose this enquiry on my patients, nevertheless I will just check whether the patient wants to go deeper in their enquiry or is just happy to find better ways to deal with their stress. This can usually be done by just changing the story and the emotions attached to the other story will disappear. Check the chapter on 'Dealing with Stress'.

Changing one's lifestyle may be the most important shift one can make in terms of health and progression into old age. Anti-aging is an incorrect term to define this process. All one is doing is optimising health as one grows old. The potential to do this is enormous and is almost entirely within each person's own hands. Very few doctors are interested in health and can advise the individual in this regard. Of course we should know much of this information anyway as a great deal is just common sense. It should be clear that junk food would create a junk body and that eating excess refined carbohydrates could lead to diabetes and obesity. We all know by now that smoking is not healthy and excess alcohol can damage the liver.

We may not be so clear about the role of toxins in the environment and how they affect our health. Much of this information is downplayed and even hidden from view. We certainly need to become more informed about water and air pollution.

Neither are most governments or big business particularly interested in health promotion. While government departments of Health should be interested in health as a priority, most money spent is used for treating diseases such as AIDS and TB. Health clinics are really 'disease' clinics and very little is being done to improve the health of individuals apart from giving drugs to treat the disease.

Disease today is expected generally to be with that person for the rest of their lives and drug taking therefore only increases with time so that by the age of 60years most individuals are taking more than 5 drugs already. Some of the drugs taken are merely treating the symptoms of other drugs.

Many people are so disempowered by being in front of their specialist that they seldom ask questions and are just too happy to take another drug. As I keep pointing out medical treatment and even investigations of any kind can be dangerous to health and is the 3rd or 4th most common cause of ill health and even death.

It is a really good idea to take personal responsibility for your health. Supporting health may mean that fewer drugs are necessary, may save you from the extra burden of surgery and even add to the length of good quality life.

Chapter 20

The story of Dr. Mary Newport and her husband is remarkable for its simplicity in helping a person with a really seriously advanced case of Alzheimer's disease recover a great deal of function. Mr. Newport started developing Alzheimer symptoms in his early 50s. Within years he deteriorated with increasing forgetfulness, could no longer be trusted to leave the house on his own, had difficulty making his own food and even eating normally.

Mary, a specialist neonatologist working with new born babies, knew something of nutrition. She knew that the drugs in use could possibly slow down the process but would not reverse any of the damage already caused or make a marked improvement in the symptoms already present. In scanning the literature to find something that could work she came across the possible use of coconut oil which becomes ketone bodies in the brain. Ketone bodies are an alternative source of energy .

The brain uses glucose as a general source of energy but it seems that in Alzheimer's disease the brain cells become resistant to insulin which is required to get the glucose into the brain cells. When insulin resistance develops outside the brain and in the body generally then this is called type 2 diabetes and this is why Alzheimer's disease is regarded by some specialists as type 3 diabetes.

Mary began feeding her husband just over 2 tablespoons of coconut oil per day. What was remarkable was the speed with which changes were noted. He described the effect as if a light was being switched on in his brain and within hours of the first dose there was already an improvement as noted when tested by independent doctors. Five days later he was smiling and starting conversations which he could not do before. His mood changed dramatically, memory returned, he could work in the garden again and as she described it 'I had my husband back again'.

He would eventually be taking the equivalent of 6 tablespoons coconut oil and while he had been taking other nutrients as well, it was not until the coconut oil was introduced that the major shift began. Dr. Delport has received hundreds of testimonials from other Alzheimer's patients who have also responded positively to coconut oil. Her story can be accessed at www.coconutketones.com

Principles of Disease Management

The principle of management arises from the following understanding:

- A human being is a complex body/ emotions/ mind/ spirit system.

- The systems functions as one complex whole.

- The system attempts constantly to maintain harmony of all its functions.

- Any disharmony is due to one of three possibilities: deficiency in function, excess in function, blockage to normal function.

- When functional disturbance continues for a prolonged period of time then a breakdown can occur. A person may complain of gastro-intestinal discomfort for 20 years without any evidence of any disease until in the 21st year a diagnosis of colitis is made with visible evidence on colonoscopy.

The principle of management is to support the deficiency, calm down the excess and remove blocks from the system. In addition one needs to identify the cause of the problem.

- Identify the cause

- Complement the systems attempts to heal

- Treat symptoms if appropriate

- Surgery may be necessary

- Psychotherapy

- Teaching lifestyle management

Identifying the causes

This is covered in Chapter 9. It is important that patients understand that the practitioner cannot remove the causes of their ill health. This is the responsibility of the person. It is frequently true also that many practitioners do not have the tools or the time to scan through the patient's history searching for causes.

This is doing the patient a disservice and often leaves the patient with the idea that the ill health has no cause or the cause is unknown and therefore unimportant. As indicated in Chapter 9 almost all the causes can fit into one of three categories i.e. genetic, environmental or emotional/mental.

While it is also true that there are no single causes every effort should be made to try and identify precipitating factors, aggravating factors and possible underlying causative factors. Practitioners have a responsibility to help patient identify as many factors as possible involved in their ill health. Symptomatic treatment only is bad medicine. Lack of time is no excuse and nor is any statement to the effect that the cause is unknown and therefore there is no point in looking for causes or trying to identify a cause.

In my experience most ill people know that something in their lifestyle has contributed to their illness, that they should be changing their diet, stop smoking, not over-eat, lose weight, deal with their stress, move from their polluted environment, drink better quality water, exercise more, drink more water, cut down on coffee and alcohol, deal more effectively with their marriage, take a holiday, do meditation regularly etc. The ill person suspects that somewhere in the above list lies part of the problem and although they don't always press their doctor to identify the causes with them they are generally disappointed that this is not discussed.

'In seeking to lengthen years of life of meaningful quality, reduction of serum cholesterol may confer a few extra weeks or months, yet pursuit of certain not esoteric but common sense lifestyles can result in greatly reduced standard mortality ratios of many present 'killer' diseases, and in the lengthening of longevity.'[1].

Complementing the system's attempts to heal.

The body/mind system is always attempting to heal itself and this is an enormously complex process but there are some common sense ideas one can have about the way this is done. In the very first instance one needs to be sure that the system has all its requirements in order that

1   Walker,Labadarios et al SAMJ. 1991

functioning is optimal. There are three basic requirements that can be identified:

- Air or oxygen
- Water
- Food and nutrients

From these basic three ingredients the system is able to maintain function and replace dying cells. All cells in the body die off in time: the skin cells every few days but even major organs are replaced every few months or years. From the air, water and food the system is able to reconstruct and replace all dying cells.

The quality of these replaced cells will obviously depend on the quality of these 3 basic ingredients. If one uses cardboard to make furniture then one has cardboard furniture no matter how sophisticated the machinery is. It takes good wood to make good furniture, but then one also does need good machinery and good workmen and a good foreman and manager to make sure that everything is used appropriately.

Many health fanatics are often surprised when they discover that they have developed cancer or than their children are more frequently ill than the family next door who seem to do all the wrong things. It points again to the complexity of who we are and that we are not just material substance or bodies but bio-energetic informational systems with spiritual components all which can become dysfunctional and lead to ill health.

I am of the opinion that ill health, so called problems and difficulties of all kinds are not exactly 'wrong' but rather part of a journey in life, an opportunity to make changes, a message from ones higher self, a correcting process of the body-mind system. When ill health happens therefore, it is not just a matter of treating the problem and removing the symptoms but recognising that there is a much bigger story here that needs attention.

The human being as indicated in previous chapters is body-emotions-mind- spirit- consciousness and matter- energy- information- quantum space and the illness is happening within that context. Treating ill health as if it is a body problem only is reductionistic thinking and does not honour and respect the 'greater anatomy' which is also involved in the ill health.

To the list above we need to therefore add the following:

- Emotional health and a quiet inner presence
- Disciplined thinking
- Spiritual centeredness

and to complete this list we must add:

- Exercise
- Meditation and time for contemplation
- Sleep and rest time

and not to forget the value of the following:

- Creative relationships
- Spending time with children and babies
- Being in the presence of wise old men and women
- Listening to the sounds of nature and being in touch with nature.
- Having an animal companion

Getting started:

Any change one makes towards health will reap benefits and even add years of extra life. Obesity for example can decrease life expectancy by about 7 years in both sexes and is one of the leading preventable causes of death in adults and children. Obesity is weighted the same in terms of ill health as excessive drinking and smoking and is expected to replace smoking as the most powerful preventable risk factor.

Some 66% of women and 33% of men are overweight in South Africa. Of special concern is the number of children now overweight. Up to 5% of boys and a staggering 25% of girls in South Africa are obese or overweight. Only the UK, Canada, USA and Mexico exceed these poor statistics.

Fat activates inflammation in the body and secretes a range of hormones. What produces all this fat is not fat intake but excessive amounts of sugar. This sugar is converted by the hormone insulin into fat. Insulin is a storage hormone and the only way that all this sugar which is not used immediately can be stored is as fat.

Aggravating the problem is the lack of exercise which would normally use up glucose for energy. People have become couch potatoes, sitting around eating junk food filled with sugar while watching TV or using their mobile phones and other instruments of communication.

Lack of exercise and excessive sugar consumption are the two major causes of ill health. I often sit with the patient and we try calculate the amount of sugar consumed per day. The average tin of Coca Cola contains 8.25 teaspoons (tsp) sugar, ginger beer 13 tsp, corn flakes 2.4 tsp, rice crispies 2.5 tsp, Honey Smacks 14 tsp, carrot cake 3 tsp per slice, muffin 4.75 tsp, sponge cake 5.5 tsp, milk chocolate bar 5.75 tsp. Adding up the sugar added to tea or coffee, cakes and sweets, breakfast cereals, jam on bread, sweetbreads of all kind, fizzy drinks, sweetened yoghurt, salad dressings, sauces of all kinds, chocolate drinks and sports drinks.

When one adds up the sugar consumed during one day, it can easily go as high as 30 tsp and often can go up to 60 tsp a day. Now that is a lot of sugar especially when the American Heart Association has set a limit of 9tsp sugar for men and 6tsp of sugar per day for women.

All the rest of the sugar consumed is turned into fat for storage. Not difficult to understand therefore that people have difficulty to lose weight without making some really drastic changes to their food choices. It is often the hidden sources of added sugar that can make all the difference.

Most foods that are 'low fat' are high sugar because without the fat the food would not taste that palatable, so sugar is added. Any processed food and junk foods will contain added sugar plus preservatives and colouring matter just adding to the load of toxins the body must deal with.

Good health becomes impossible if people continue to make poor food choices.

A 2015 study conducted by the journal Frontiers in Nutrition concluded that a diet that is vegetarian five days a week and includes meat just two days a week would reduce greenhouse-gas emissions and water and land use by about 45 percent.

It appears that a healthy diet is one of the best ways to reduce elevated blood pressure. An eating plan called the Dietary Approaches to Stop Hypertension (DASH) diet – which includes lots of fruits, vegetables, nuts, legumes and low-fat dairy products and limits meat, sweets, fats and salt – is a viable way to prevent and treat high blood pressure, according to recent research. The DASH diet is also rich in magnesium, potassium, protein and fibre.

• It is often suggested that drug use is cheaper than life style interventions. In a study published in 2006[2] it was shown that the drug Metformin might delay onset of diabetes by three years, while diet and exercise change delays it by 11 years. There would also be major cost savings in the diet and exercise regimes.

• In another study[3] involving obese and overweight people with diabetes or insulin resistance there was a 50% reversal of insulin resistance and diabetes after only 3 weeks when placed on a high fibre, low-fat diet, combined with 45-60 minutes of exercise on a treadmill each day. There was even no restriction on the amount of food eaten.

There is plenty evidence to suggest that good food choices and exercise are generally better options to improve health than drugs.

So by far the most important decision one needs to make with your Integrative doctor is around the right food choices for your special needs. My general suggestion is the following:

• Elimination diet: This is basically a test diet to check for food intolerances. It excludes all dairy, all gluten foods, all preservatives and colouring matter, all junk foods and any other food the child or adult has a problem with. The diet should continue for 3 to 4 weeks and then add back one item of food every 5 days and check the person's reaction to the food added back. I prefer this approach than doing blood tests.

• My cleansing diet for one month. This is basically a vegetarian diet with some fruit and nuts in the morning for breakfast, any raw vegetables as a salad for lunch and cooked vegetables for supper.

2   Wylie-Rosett et al Lifestyle Intervention to prevent diabetes: Intensive and cost effective. Current Opinion in Lipidology.17 (1); 2006: 37-44

3   Christian et al Effect of a short term diet and exercise intervention on oxidative stress, inflammation, MMP-9 and Monocyte Chem- tactic activity in men with Metabolic syndrome factors. Journal of Applied Physiology 2006;100:1657-65

Olive oil, coconut oil, sesame paste (tahini) and sea salt can be added freely. Sprouts are good.

• Mediterranean diet is my suggested basic healthy diet for maintenance. It should include lots of farm fresh vegetables and fruit, organic if possible with free-range meat, chicken and eggs a few times per week, fish 2-3 times per week, fermented foods, nuts and seeds and sprouts. A glass or two of red wine is okay for some people but alcohol is a liver poison so this should not be a daily intake. Grains are problematic and should be carefully assessed by each individual. Wheat is no longer a good food and all grains have generally been stored over time requiring fumigation to prevent rot and fungus growth. Rye is better if one can tolerate gluten otherwise gluten free choice is essential.

• Banting/ketogenic diet: These to my mind are specialised diets that help under certain circumstances. The diet is the best way to lose weight quickly for most individuals. A strict ketogenic diet is probably the best way to control epilepsy and is also shown to work for people with brain cancer. I generally don't recommend diets long term that require counting, measuring and excessive restrictions nevertheless these diets can make major shifts in disease management and help weight reduction rapidly.

• Paleo diet or the Hunter-gatherers diet: This diet makes some sense because it returns us back to the diet that our ancestors ate. Foods are fresh and in season and include meat, fish, vegetables and some fruit. Clearly all processed and junk foods are excluded.

There are a range of other diets which claim to help. Keep it simple and don't become fanatical about any diet. Generally it is common sense and we all know what good food looks like. Processed food generally means that all goodness has been removed, over-heated, destroying much of its rich diversity of nutrients, poor quality food often used, synthetic vitamins with poor nutritional status added, other chemicals added to preserve the food and then subjected to varying lengths of storage with further deterioration of quality.

Exercise and stress management are the other legs of the stool of health management. With right food choices, exercise and stress management in place everyone should notice some improvement in health. It really is as simple as that. Unfortunately the majority of doctors can't help you in this department. lifestyle management is generally not even stressed in medical school, the doctor is not following healthy choices and so does not want to even talk about the subject and it would complicate his consulting time.

Much easier to take out a prescription pad and write a prescription for drugs. Everyone is happy. The doctor can move you on and vey often people do not want to be confronted with something they actually know already or don't want to make decisions that will take away those foods that they find most enjoyable which are the junk and processed foods.

First step in management: Right food choices, exercise and stress management.

Is there any evidence that lifestyle changes really work or is it just some fairy story of health fanatics? Well, the American Heart Association, the National Heart, Lung and Blood Institute all recommend lifestyle changes as a primary approach to cholesterol lowering for example.

While statins are often prescribed for both primary and secondary prevention as a primary treatment to prevent heart attacks, this is only because most doctors don't want to talk about lifestyle and generally feel more secure in prescribing drugs. Nevertheless their own associations do suggest lifestyle changes as a primary approach to a range of diseases including cardiovascular disease, mild to moderate hypertension and diabetes prevention.

Evidence that this basic approach is effective when faithfully followed is decisive. Studies such as the 'Lyon-Diet Heart Study'[4] have shown that a Mediterranean diet based on specific food changes lowers the risk of heart attack in high risk individuals by as much as 70%.[5]

4   de Lorgeril M, Salen P, Martin J-L, et al.
      Mediterranean diet, traditional risk factors, and the
      rate of cardiovascular complications after myocardial
      infarction. Final report of the Lyon Diet Heart Study.
      Circulation 1999;99:779-85.
5   Singh RB, Dubnov G, Niaz MA, et al. Effect of an
      Indo-Mediterranean diet on progression of coronary
      artery disease in high risk patients
      (Indo-Mediterranean Diet Heart Study): a
      randomised single-blind trial. Lancet 2002;360:1455

Studies by Ornish and colleagues[6] have shown that a vegetarian diet can actually reverse the narrowing of the coronary arteries as detected with angiographic recordings.

The 'Dietary Approaches to Stop Hypertension' (DASH) studies[7] have shown that a mostly plant-based diet with low- or non-fat dairy can lower stage 1 blood pressure as effectively as drugs.

The 'Diabetes Prevention Program'[8] showed that lifestyle was twice as effective as the drug metformin in preventing diabetes in high-risk individuals, reducing its occurrence by 58 percent. So the drug did worked. Compared to placebo, in terms of the percentage of people developing diabetes within the four-year study period, fewer people in the drug group developed diabetes.

But diet and exercise alone worked better. The lifestyle intervention reduced diabetes incidence by 58 %, compared to only 31% with the drug. The lifestyle intervention was significantly more effective than the drug, and had fewer side effects. More than three quarters of those on the drug reported gastrointestinal symptoms, though there was more muscle soreness reported in the lifestyle group, on account of them actually exercising.

The 'Portfolio Study'[9], proved the principle that diet can lower LDL cholesterol as effectively as statin drugs.

6   Ornish D, Scherwitz LW, Billings JH, et al. Intensive lifestyle changes for reversal of coronary heart disease. JAMA 1998; 280: 2001-7.

7   Moore TJ et al DASH (Dietary Approaches to stop Hypertension) is effective treatment for stage 1 isolated systolic hypertension. Hyp- tension. 2001;38(2):155

8   Knowler WC et al Reduction in the incidence of type 2 diabetes with lifestyle intervention or metformin. NEJM 2002;346(6):393-403

9   Jenkins D et al Direct comparison of a dietary portfolio of cholesterol-lowering foods with a statin in hypercholesterolemic participants. Am J Clinical Nutrition 2005;81(2):380-387

So, there is nothing at all radical about using lifestyle changes to improve health, reduce ill health and even turn ill health and disease back to much better health without the use of drugs or to reduce the amount of drugs being taken.

Eighty percent of heart attacks in men are preventable by changes in lifestyle, according to research conducted at the Karolinska Institute. The study, published in the Journal of the American College of Cardiology, surveyed data on over 20,000 Swedish men aged 45-79, who were tracked from 1997 to 2009.

The team isolated five aspects of a healthy lifestyle - eating a healthy diet, staying in good shape, exercising regularly, staying away from tobacco and controlling alcohol intake - and surveyed the men on their lifestyles.

Based on the findings of the study, the team estimated that practicing the five healthy behaviors could prevent nearly 80 percent of first time heart attacks in men.

'It is not surprising that healthy lifestyle choices would lead to a reduction in heart attacks,' said Agneta Akesson, the lead researcher for the study. 'What is surprising is how drastically the risk dropped due to these factors.'

Why are these authors surprised and not surprised at the same time? Firstly, we know that heart disease; diabetes and many cancers were very much less common 100 years ago. Even Autoimmune disease and allergies were much less common than they are today. Clearly genetics cannot be blamed because of the short interval in which these shifts in chronic disease have happened.

It also means that these chronic diseases often called chronic diseases of lifestyle can be shifted and are not a consequence of modern society but more a consequence of choices people make. It also suggests that low rates of these diseases can be attained without the use of drugs. Using drugs is often an easy way out both for doctors and their patients who don't want to take responsibility for making lifestyle changes.[10]

10   Willett W. C. Balancing Lifestyle and Genom- ics Research for Disease Prevention. Science. 2002; 296:695–98

Diabetes was almost unknown in China 30 years ago and now there are millions of people with prediabetes and diabetes. lifestyle changes are all modifiable factors that everyone has the ability of changing. Some recent studies have pointed to the astonishing ability of the body to shift back to normal. In type 2 diabetes even after one week of a very restricted diet (800calories) fasting glucose normalised, insulin suppression of liver glucose output improved and maximal insulin response became normal at 8 weeks.

Normalization of pancreatic beta cell function and insulin sensitivity was achieved by dietary energy restriction alone within 8 weeks.[11] What was a revelation to me was the fact that pancreatic hormonal insulin function could actually return to normal function so rapidly suggesting that these cells secreting insulin had not actually 'died' but had just gone to sleep from overuse i.e. exhaustion. The longer the diabetes 2 had been present the less normality was achieved, nevertheless many long term DM2 still responded positively.

This is also called the Newcastle Diet and has spawned a range of different ways to achieve this goal over the long term. The 5 + 2 Diet for example allows free food choices for 5 days in the week and then 2 days of low calorie diet. Others have tried keeping the eating programme to 8 hours only during the day and then a long fast from the early evening meal, no breakfast apart from coffee or tea and then an early lunch and supper.

All these approaches seem to work, suggesting the enormous possibilities of helping people come back to good health without the needs for drugs.

Heart disease and diabetes are reversible with lifestyle changes. No drugs required.

The Merck Manual (17th edition, pp. 2591-2592) essentially states that up to 90% of cancer is preventable: 'Environmental or nutritional factors probably account for up to 90% of human cancers. These factors

---

11   Lim et al Reversal of type 2 diabetes: normalization of
      beta cell function in association with decreased
      pancreas and liver triacylglycerol. Diabetologia
      2011;54(10):2506-14

include smoking, diet, and exposure to sunlight, chemicals, and drugs. Genetic, viral, and radiation factors may cause the rest.'

The biggest myth of modern medicine is that the increase in average human lifespan in the last hundred years is primarily due to doctors and drugs. In fact, the increased lifespan is due primarily to the wealth effect (as nations become wealthier, lifespan increases) and public health measures such as better sanitation, better protection from the elements (better housing), better nutrition, greater access to clean water, etc.

Modern medicine has played a role, but that role is modest compared to social, cultural, economic, and political factors.

The decline in mortality from infectious diseases has been a major reason for people living longer. These infectious diseases declined not primarily due to vaccination but due mainly to improved sanitation, improved nutrition, reduced exposure to infection because of better housing, and better water supply and quality. When these conditions deteriorate then infectious diseases and food poisoning become a major problem. These improvements were happening already during the 19th century, while modern medical treatment and vaccinations only appeared during the 20th century.[12]

The introduction of antibiotics in the late 1940s and early 1950s played a much smaller role in the increase in lifespan in the last hundred years than is commonly believed. The death rates from infectious diseases had already fallen to low levels by the time that antibiotics were introduced.

By 1950, when effective antitubercular drugs first became widely available, the death rate from tuberculosis, the major infectious disease of young adults, had already fallen to a small fraction of what it had been in the nineteenth century.[13]

12 Sagan, Leonard. The Health of Nations: True Causes of Sickness and Well-being, New York: Basic Books, 1987, p. 64.

13 McKinlay, J. B., and McKinlay, S. M. "The Questionable Contribution of Medical Meas- ures to the Decline of Mortality in the United States in the Twentieth Century," Millbank Memorial Fund Quarterly (Summer), pp. 405-428, 1977

I have emphasised the benefits of exercise in Chapter 19 on lifestyle management but in writing this chapter I came across a Time article of September 19th 2016 about the work of Dr Mark Tarnopolsky, a genetic metabolic neurologist. He made the following statements about his research on exercise;

'But as time goes on, paper after paper shows that the most effective, potent way that we can improve quality of life and duration of life is exercise.

'Going for a run is going to improve your skin health, your eye health, your gonadal health' and finally he continues

'If there was a drug that could do for human health everything that exercise can, it would likely be the most valuable pharmaceutical ever developed.'

It seems that only 20% of Americans get the recommended 150 minutes of strength and cardiovascular physical activity per week, more than half of all baby boomers report doing no exercise whatsoever, and 80.2 million Americans over age 6 are entirely inactive.

Hopefully those reading this book will have got the message by now about lifestyle management and why it is so much more important than taking drugs.

I have perhaps laboured the need for lifestyle changes but I have come to the conclusion over the years that both the lay public and the medical establishment have tended to dismiss lifestyle as significant compared to the use of drugs and even surgery.

In the chapter on the placebo response I have mentioned studies that even when surgery was compared to sham surgery (incisions made and stitched but no further surgery performed) that the people having the sham surgery still responded as if real surgery was performed. Sham surgery has helped not only in cases of arthritis of the knees but also when sham surgery was performed for angina due to narrowing of the coronary arteries.

So just in case you think I made a mistake here, let me repeat this study in which a group of patients with angina (pain due to heart vessel narrowing) were divided into two groups. The one group had a regular procedure performed for this condition and the other group only had a skin incision plus stitches and nothing further, yet both groups responded positively. This operation was soon abandoned. Perhaps other operations should be subject to this kind of study.

lifestyle changes should always be the number one approach to any ill health or disease.

Second step: Optimising nutrient status:

As indicated in previous chapters, everyone is nutrient deficient. Any nutrient deficiency means that the systems in the body are under stress and will not be functioning at their optimum. Important to keep in mind that it is the nutrients from food that make life possible. The body is never deficient in drugs.

Long before drugs are prescribed the doctor should first be talking about lifestyle changes, then prescribing nutrients required to improve function. There is not a single function in the body that does not need nutrients for moment-to-moment functionality.

Nutrients are used up constantly for digestion, exercise, liver detoxification, brain function, heart, kidney, adrenals and a myriad of other functions in the body. Cell membranes must be healthy, stomach acid is constantly being replenished and used up in the digestive process, enzymes are needed all over the body etc. The turnover of nutrients is enormous and is even critical during the early years of growing up but also as one ages.

With such an enormous nutritional requirements by the body, how does one decide then what to take as extra nutrition assuming that one has already made some good food choices, and removed all junk food.

These are my suggestions:

• Vitamin D3 between 3000IU and 5000IU per day depending on the season and colour of ones skin. The darker the skin the less sun penetration and therefore the less vitamin D is produced in the body. The body cannot make vitamin D without sun exposure. Vitamin D has a range of important functions and includes genetic health.

• Omega 3 either as fish oil or krill oil. This is essential for cell membrane health and decreasing the inflammation in the body.

• A good quality mineral/trace mineral and vitamin combination. I prefer this in ionic form, which usually means a liquid preparation.

That's a really good start provided of course that lifestyle changes are included with better food choices, some simple exercises every day and dealing with stress. Please read my chapter on stress management.

Perhaps add some meditation or just sitting quietly with deep breathing and relaxing music. Spending time chatting to your dog or cat is also a useful way of relaxing by increasing oxytocin levels in the blood.

The majority of people even with more serious chronic diseases will respond positively to these very simple changes. If you are already taking drugs then you may need to consult with your doctor and tell him what you are doing because it may become necessary to reduce the drug dosage, sometimes dramatically. Don't be surprised if there are major shifts in the way you feel.

Aggravation of symptoms during the first 7 to 10 days

During the first week or 10 days of amy serious changes to food sources it is possible that you may feel worse. This is due to the fact that the body will now begin a healing process and toxins come out of the fat tissue especially if weight reduction happens. People complain of headaches, tiredness, brain fog, muscle aches and pains, nausea and even diarrhoea. All this is quite a normal response to the cleansing diet for the first month. Symptoms should disappear after a few days.

Going to the next level:

Keep in mind that lifestyle changes are still the most important part of starting to become healthier and drug free and then add the basics described above. As indicate just doing the above i.e. lifestyle changes plus the few remedies suggested is enough to prevent a whole range of ill health and disease but will also turn around cardiovascular disease including angina, diabetes, many autoimmune diseases and almost any other disease you may have. It can help reduce symptoms and even reduce the need for many drugs and avoid surgery.

Despite the above there are many reasons for lack of improvement or insufficient progress of the ill health towards better health.

- Stress factors not being addressed deep enough.
- Specific nutrients required in higher doses because of certain genetic traits.
- Toxins blocking the system and preventing health.
- Disease has progressed too far for a return of function to normal.

- Excess metals in the body such as mercury, lead, aluminum.

- Poor sleep patterns.

- Avoiding some lifestyle changes such as smoking habit, excess alcohol, and addictions.

- Excessive reliance on drugs for symptomatic control.

Each one of these factors needs to be addressed, as they can be a major block to better health. Help may be required to get passed these blocks. You may by now be thinking 'what about my disease, when are we going to address this'. Treating the 'disease' without paying attention to lifestyle management, removing causes and managing the underlying dysfunctions makes no sense to any Integrative doctor. Real healing is not possible if these other factors are not central to management.

All diseases are 'end point' problems and behind the disease is a range of dysfunctions, which are common to them all. Trying to treat the disease using drugs without any attempt to correct lifestyle and dealing with the underlying dysfunction will not heal the problem. Some of the underlying dysfunctions include the following:

- Leaky gut

- Insulin resistance

- Methylation disturbance

- Hormonal deregulations involving thyroid, adrenals, sex hormones, melatonin

- Adrenal fatigue

- Acid-base imbalance

- Immune system deregulation

- Gut flora disturbances

- Low stomach acid

- Cell membrane dysfunction

- Sleep disturbances

- An inflamed brain

- Inflammation generally

- Neurotransmitter problems
- Mitochondrial disturbances
- Ageing processes
- Enzyme blocks
- Small intestine bacterial overgrowth (SIBO)
- Fatty liver- alcoholic and non alcoholic
- Poor hydration
- Auto-immune reactions
- Hypothalamic-pituitary axis disturbances
- Obesity
- Metabolic disturbance

These are just some of the underlying disturbances behind all disease. The longer a disturbance is present, the more systems and disturbances become involved until eventually evidence of a disease becomes obvious. Behind every disease, even those with the same name, the underlying group of dysfunctions will not be exactly the same and even the disease with the same name will therefore have a range of different presentations regarding symptoms and signs.

Treating the disease with drugs which focus on the disease as an entity cannot possibly be curative for the simple reason that the range of underlying dysfunctions are not corrected. Here are some examples of what I mean:

Treating ear infections with antibiotics.

While it may seem obvious that bacteria or virus may be the cause, the fact is that no microorganism can really cause a problem unless the immune system is compromised. So behind that ear infection is an immune system that needs support. The infection is a great way to activate the immune system but too often doctors give antibiotics, which shuts down the process and prevents a good activation of the immune system. A second antibiotic will only weaken the immune response even more, leading to a history of recurrent ear infections.

Treating cancer by removing the cancer and then using chemotherapy.

Cancer can take 20 years to slowly develop. All this time the body's anticancer mechanisms are slowly becoming weakened by poor diet, cancer producing toxins, stress, mitochondrial dysfunction, free radical damage etc. Removing the cancer and treating with chemotherapy or radiotherapy does very little to the underlying problem, which remains, and any secondary's, which have escaped the destructive effect of the treatment, can now slowly grow again to cause problems.

Fixing the broken part of a car without doing a tune-up is really poor workmanship. Removing the cancer and treating with chemotherapy without considering lifestyle changes and trying to optimize healthy function is poor medical practice.

Using anti-inflammatory drugs to treat inflammation such as acute injuries or more serious chronic diseases such as rheumatoid arthritis.

Acute inflammation is the way the body heals injury. It is the natural response to any injury. Using anti-inflammatory drugs therefore make no sense to an Integrative doctor. There are natural ways to support the body's inflammatory process and optimize its efficiency so that healing moves easily and harmoniously towards good, strong repair.

But what about chronic inflammation which is regarded as a serious problem and the underlying cause of much ill health including heart disease and neurodegenerative conditions such as Parkinson's disease and Multiple sclerosis. Inflammation should never become chronic.

There are very efficient control mechanisms in place that will generally prevent this from happening. Using anti-inflammatory medication to try and shut down the inflammation is band-aid medicine. The anti-inflammatory drugs have no intelligence but do what they are meant to do without taking into account the intelligence of the system and the underlying dysfunctional processes that have caused the chronic ongoing inflammation.

Are natural anti-inflammatory products not doing the same thing? Omega 3, curcumin, enzymes are all used by integrative doctors when inflammation is present and they are often described as anti-inflammatory agents. It is important to keep in mind that the body has its own inflammatory and anti-inflammatory promoters.

Inflammation is a highly intelligent, complex and coordinated process. Natural products are themselves extremely complex unlike the simple chemical drugs produced by Pharmaceutical companies. While some of these natural products may be classified as anti-inflammatory, they are generally much more complex and can also be called anti-oxidant, anticancer, cell membrane support, immune system balancing and many other functions including supplying vitamins, minerals, trace minerals and other important nutrients. It would therefore be wrong to think of them as one would drugs. So a natural anti-inflammatory product has many other functions, which support health unlike drugs and work much closer to the body's own anti-inflammatory processes. They therefore seldom cause serious side effects.

Attempting to treat Parkinson's disease with drugs.

Parkinson's disease is a problem of deficient dopamine in the brain so that drugs attempt to increase dopamine levels in different ways. They may increase dopamine, mimic dopamine or prevent the breakdown of dopamine thus increasing the level in the brain. It does make some sense doing all these things so why is the treatment only symptomatic and never cures anyone with Parkinson's disease.

The problem again is that doctors are not dealing with the underlying causes (food choices, stress, nutritional deficiencies, toxins etc.) and the consequent dysfunction, which arises as a result of these causes. Each Parkinson's case is unique and while the 'end point' is similar, the underlying causes and dysfunction are unique to that patient.

Integrative doctors will discuss lifestyle and then suggest the various options to optimize healthy functions and slowly watch what the body can do to heal itself. The system really wants to heal.

Treating heart disease with stents.

Heart disease was almost unknown 100 years ago and now is the number one killer. I think it is generally agreed by everyone, even cardiologists that lifestyle management is number one management and reversal of the coronary artery narrowing is possible just by changing lifestyle. Stents are only required in an acute emergency. So why are stents so easily inserted?

Here again we see the powerful mindset around immediate resolving of a problem even though there are serious risks involved including death. Changing lifestyle is often resisted and stents and drug medication chosen instead. I do blame the medical profession however for not spending more time in providing patients with the various options available. The truth is that few cardiologists even bother to check the results of diet changes, exercise and stress management and seldom emphasize these strategies.

Apart from lifestyle there are some really good nutritional supplements for cardio-vascular problems including garlic, hawthorn, vitamin E and C, magnesium, taurine, coenzyme Q10 and carnitine.

Treating diabetes with insulin.

Insulin may be essential in type 1 diabetes but type 2 diabetes is generally a lifestyle management problem and due to poor food choices and the development of insulin resistance. Adding insulin when insulin resistance is present will not improve the condition over the long term. Diabetes type 2 can be easily reversed especially in the early stages by better food choices and nutrients that support function.

Treating children with attention problems with Ritalin.

Few children actually need to be given drugs so early in their life. Just as doctors don't like to spend time with patients talking about lifestyle changes, teachers and parents also want quick fixes and drugs become the easy way out. Remove junk food especially the up and down swings of sugar loading and watch behavior change. Add some omega 3, Evening Primrose oil, vitamin D, the herbs bacopa, rhodiola, 5-hydroxy tryptophan and tyrosine for the next level of treatment.

Treating insomnia with synthetic drugs.

These can be seriously addicting and should seldom be used. There are a range of natural products that can be taken together, but also remember to check out the underlying factors preventing sleep.

In all these examples powerful synthetic drugs are used to treat an end point problem without dealing with the underlying metabolic disturbances. The aim is really to try to control the symptoms and leave the person generally with the need to take drugs for the rest of their life. With cancer, as already indicated, the removal of the cancer and using chemotherapy leaves the underlying metabolic dysfunction behind.

Treat symptoms of disease with drugs

Or

Support healthy functions by lifestyle changes and optimising function.

The principles of management include the following:

- Better lifestyle choices

- Remove toxins

- Optimize nutrient status

- Check for dysfunctionality of systems

- Treat disease if appropriate using least invasive and least dangerous options.

Better lifestyle choices have already been discussed in this chapter and many other chapters in this book.

Removing toxins and metals from the body

Toxins and metals can interfere with any management protocol including the use of drugs so that every effort should be made to remove them.

Any fasting will help a great deal to get the toxins out. Why one feels unwell for the first day or two is that the toxins come out of the storage areas into the blood on their way to the liver for removal. Sweating is the best way to eliminate toxins as most toxins are stored in the fatty and subcutaneous tissues close to the surface of the body and do not need to go through the blood and liver pathway when sweated out.

Other methods to eliminate toxins and metals include the use of zeolite (volcanic ash), chlorophyll containing products such as spirulina, chlorella, barley green and various chelation processes using EDTA and DMSA.

Supporting liver function and dealing with leaky gut are all essential to prevent more toxins entering and to make sure that the most important organ of detoxification, the liver, is functioning at its optimum best.

Optimising nutrient status

Everyone has nutrient deficiencies and very few people are functioning at their optimum possibilities. In addition there is a need for a constant supply of nutrients. Just like the heart, none of the systems in the body ever stop working unless the person is dead. Even in sleep the body is working to retune, remove toxins and build up energy supply before the person wakes up and starts activities again.

For this reason I always suggest people start with Vitamin D, Omega 3 and a vitamin mineral/trace mineral supplement. That's a good start. I have never come across anyone with really robust levels of vitamin D and omega 3 is a great anti-inflammatory and the fatty acids rebalance the omega3 to 6 ratios, which is generally abnormal in most people. I love adding coconut oil to my basic formula because the fatty acids supply ketones for brain function and have been shown to reverse brain degeneration. Coconut oil also has antifungal properties, which will treat any candida around in the gastro-intestinal tract.

Withdraw any non-essential drugs

In my experience a good 25% or more of the symptoms and signs I see in my practice are due to the side effects of drugs. Many of the drugs given are to treat the side effects of other drugs and not really due to the disease. Doctors clearly oversubscribe rather than discuss lifestyle changes with their patient. Drug prescribing is easy, quick, makes money and even patients often insist on getting a drug to treat the symptoms.

Here we are discussing health promotion and getting off drugs is highly recommended. Some drugs are easily stopped while others should only be stopped with the help of your practitioner. There are many natural approaches which can be used instead of drugs but don't expect your conventional medical practitioner to know much about these approaches.

Everyone has a range of dysfunctions and stress factors, but start with the gastrointestinal area.

One of the key areas of disturbances is the gastro-intestinal area and probably why changing the diet can make such a big difference. In the elderly, stomach acid is often too low. In children food intolerance is a major problem and this includes gluten and milk intolerance but any other food may also be a problem. Over time this can lead to leaky gut followed by a range of autoimmune disturbances.

Apart from elimination diets, the Integrative doctor may suggest pancreatic enzymes to help digestion, Betaine hydrochloride to deal with low acidity, probiotics and prebiotics, glutamine or one of my favourites for leaky gut, colostrum. Not to forget adding extra fibre especially if constipation is present and to eliminate toxins present in the bowel.

I know of a number of Integrative Psychiatrists who start their management of psychiatric disorders by focusing on the gastro-intestinal area. This is not surprising as the Gut-Brain connection is well known and it is estimated that 90% of the serotonin in the body is made in the gastrointestinal area.

No need to fill up all the holes

Just with the above information one can go a really long way in dealing with and improving most chronic ill health. Yes, I really mean that. I really believe that most any disease will respond 20-80% just with the above information i.e. lifestyle changes plus adding vitamin D, omega 3 and a good vitamin, mineral supplement plus dealing with the intestinal tract and optimising its function plus removing unnecessary drugs. The next phase may require more specialised under standing and help.

Here are some examples of what I mean.

• If the patient is complaining of severe tiredness and lack of energy then consider supporting mitochondrial function with coenzyme Q10, carnitine and D-Ribose.

• Hormonal disturbances. Always consider bio-identical hormones rather than synthetic non-identical hormones or hormones derived from horses urine.

• Diabetes type 2 does not require drugs. It is a metabolic problem due to excess refined carbohydrates especially sugar. The herbal extract Berberine works just as well as metformin with fewer side effects.

• Thyroid hormone deficiency is a major problem. Even if the thyroid hormone profile is within the low normal level but the patient has symptoms of low thyroid function, they should be given a trial of thyroid hormone. Keep in mind though that eltroxin which is T4 must be changed to T3 which is the active form of the hormone and that this conversion from T4 to T3 requires a specific enzyme, which becomes deficient as we age. This means that many people are being told that their hormonal status is normal based on a T4 measurement only when in fact they also need to take T3 together with the T4.

• Sleep is essential for health. Drugs are not a good idea, as they do not produce a normal sleep cycle. Natural remedies should be tried including valerian, 5-HTP, hops, L-theanine, lavender and even medicinal cannabis can help in serious cases.

• Inflammation is a major underlying cause of many chronic diseases. Elimination diet, Mediterranean diet, exercise are all part of management and should also include weight reduction. Deal with the leaky gut if present. Omega 3, curcumin, Boswellia, green tea, colostrum, ginger, low dose naltrexone, and probiotics can all help to reduce inflammation.

• Methylation cycle support. This is a very important detoxification cycle often found dysfunctional in many conditions such as autism, cardiovascular disease, Parkinson's disease and many other neurodegenerative conditions. Check for homocysteine levels and if abnormally high then consider giving a combination of folic acid, B12, B6, TMG, Betaine.

Anti Ageing

I prefer to use the words 'ageing well' rather than anti-ageing. What one is trying to do is not reverse ageing but to optimize health as one ages. The potential is enormous because as suggested over and over again, very few people are functioning at their optimum but in fact far below their optimum functionality.

As I age I have been taking more and more supplements especially those referred to as 'adaptogens'. This latter group of herbal products helps the body to adapt to stress without over stimulating and just supporting. They can be taken long term and seldom produce side effects.

Adaptogens include the following: Ashwaganda, Rhodiola, Ginseng (Asian, Siberian, American), Astragalus, some mushrooms (cordyceps, rheishi), Eleutherococcus, Schisandra, Shilajit.

Vitamin D, omega 3, vitamin K, vitamin C, vitamin E, and vitamin Bs are all essential and should be added even if one has a good diet. Keep in mind that we are talking about optimising the nutritional status. As one ages all metabolic functions become problematic and require extra nutrients. Good food choices alone would not be sufficient to optimise functions.

Take weekend holidays from nutrients but extra nutrients, sometimes even in high doses, are required.

Brom's rules around management

In my teaching to Health practitioners I refer constantly to these following rules:

1: Every case is unique, no matter what the name of the disease is.

You are always dealing with unique genetic background, unique combination of causes, unique responses of systems and unique intelligence trying to deal with the stress within the system.

2: Don't get caught up in the diagnosis of the disease.

It is the underlying dysfunction which is important rather than the disease.

3: Everyone has a range of dysfunctions and stress factors.

These are unique to that person.

4: No one is functioning at optimum levels even when healthy.

5: Keep it simple - the body wants to heal.

Think of removing the pressure within the system, ie stress, food choices, toxins, and then think what can be added to support health.

6: Don't need to fill up all the holes.

Just one or two changes can shift everything. The body systems want to heal and will do so rapidly if given the opportunity .

7: Everyone has some vitamin and mineral deficiencies

The most common is probably vitamin D. Other important deficiencies are magnesium, iodine, vitamin C, B vitamins, zinc.

8: Remove as many drugs as you can. Drugs intefere with function and force the body to use pathways that may not be optimum .

9: When healing happens it is not a cause-effect phenomenon, but holographic.

As indicated in other chapter, living systems do not function in straight lines but follow very complex pathways that are interactive and entangled.

10: The Healer and patient are also entangled in their interaction.

The electromagnetic recording of the heart for example extends outwardly into the environment even up to a metre away from the body.

11: Ill health is not meant to be a problem but part of the journey of life we are all on.

Keep it simple with the knowledge that the innate healing capacity of the body wants to heal itself. It knows what to do and only requires some help along the way.

Chapter 21

It was the evening before I was to start my teaching course and this was also the second day of my excruciating back pain. It was so severe that if I lay down in bed I could not get out of the bed so I had resorted to sitting in a reclining chair used in my clinic downstairs for acupuncture. This particular chair would at the press of a button lift the body right up into a semi-standing position that made it possible for me to at least get to the toilet if necessary and then to get into a semi- horizontal position to sleep.

The problem was that my teaching the next day included one student coming from overseas to my course in Integrative medicine. There was no way I could cancel the course at this late stage. Medical doctors had given up a number of days to attend and some were already in B & B's within walking distance of my home.

I was feeling quite desperate. For the first time in probably 20 years I decided to take a powerful pain pill. That was at about 9 pm. By 4 am in the morning there was no change and the pain was extreme with any movement. Sitting and teaching would have been impossible.

So I did what perhaps most people in this kind of situation might consider doing and that is prayed. I prayed to God, to Great Mystery explaining my predicament and why I needed help to get rid of the pain, which was making life impossibly difficult. When I stopped praying and lay back exhausted I suddenly heard this voice in my head saying, 'ask what love is saying to you'.

What love is saying! You mean the pain in my back is the voice of love. Yes was the reply. I was astonished at that thought and it seemed to strike some really deep core inside my consciousness. It was as if I suddenly knew that our ill health and my back pain were not haphazard occurrences but meaningful and part of my journey in life. With this thought every cell in my body seem to go into a deep relaxation and acceptance around the idea that it was love talking to me through the pain. I fell into a deep sleep and awoke free of pain.

The pain was almost 90% gone all of the next day and continued to improve over the 4 days of the teaching course allowing me to move, sit and teach.

Do we Need God for Healing?

As a doctor one often hears similar stories of miraculous healing in animals, humans and even plants. There are also stories of apparent synchronicity of events that seem miraculous in the way they have emerged. You think of phoning someone you have not spoken to for months or even years and as you walk towards the phone, that person telephones you. You go on holiday in another country and you bump into someone from your school while visiting some remote village in the jungle where very few foreigners visit. It seems almost as if this meeting with your old school buddy is not by chance and slowly as the two of you talk it becomes obvious why this meeting is happening.

Rupert Sheldrake has written about his research on dogs who seemed to know when their master was coming home even when the return times were changed from day to day, including the method of transport. In another book he examined the way that people knew when they were being stared at and would turn around and look at the person staring at them.

As he points out, there is no science at present to explain this phenomenon and if these simple stories are true and can be verified by a few other scientists then everything we know about Newtonian reductionistic science needs to be reviewed, at least with regard to living systems. That dogs know when their owner is coming home, pigeons and monarch butterflies homing ability, the organization skills of termites, people that know when they are being stared at, the power of prayer, the astonishing skills of some autistic children, mental telepathy and many other skills demonstrated by living systems, all these phenomenon which don't fit into classic mechanistic theories and explanations suggest that living systems don't react or respond according to reductionistic science as understood today.

The general belief in reductionism (reducing everything to its most basic forms) that seems to have gripped modern scientists has oversimplified life and taken the mystery away leaving it to the poets and artists to remind us of a part of our lives that does seem to walk alongside this very objective and material world.

'Mechanists have always feared, and still fear that to admit the reality of anything 'mysterious' or 'mystical' in the realm of life would be to abandon the hard-won certainties of science.'[1]

I also know that in my most creative writing there is a shared relationship with another part of my mind. I call this a relationship between the thinking conscious mind and the knowing unconscious mind. The word unconscious is perhaps inappropriate because that part of the mind is actually more conscious that the apparently consciousness mind.

A better way to think about this distinction is from a functional perspective. There is the 'thinking mind' and another part of the mind that does not think but appears to 'know'. This knowing is not linear but appears to be beyond time and space.

Thinking mind and knowing mind

Intuition reaches into this beyond time and space dimension. My logical thinking mind can ask a question to this knowing mind and can wait for the intuitive impulse which is usually translated into thought by the thinking mind. An example of this is my story above of my very serious back pain. All my logical mind could eventually do when it had exhausted all options and nothing was working was to pray.

Prayer is the ultimate acknowledgement of the logical thinking mind eventually realising that it is impotent in the face of the present challenge and now 'asks' for help for itself or another. In that moment a response arises. It is not a logical thinking process because that has 'given up' and allowed another part of the mind to respond. That response was not just a message interpreted by the thinking mind as an intuitive impulse but came with a remarkable healing of my back pain.

What we call unconscious is only not conscious to the thinking part of the mind but appears to have information, knowingness and wisdom that are not directly available to my thinking 'conscious' mind. There is often a response from this unconscious part of Self in the form of a healing, money appearing, job offer, meeting a person etc. in a most synchronize and spontaneous way. Something the logical, thinking mind could not have planned.

1   Sheldrake T Seven Experiments that could change the world. 2002. Park Street Press. P5

The logical thinking mind would love to be involved but eventually recognizes its impotence and inability to transcend itself , lets go, relaxes and discovers in this letting go an inner peace appears. This is also what happens in meditation when the meditator is able to step back from thought and discovers the quiet place just below thinking.

From a functional perspective then I separate mind into two parts. First there is the conscious logical, linear mind and then there is that part of the mind that is not directly available to my conscious mind and yet feeds me with information via the bridge of intuition.

These two parts of the mind do work together but it is the thinking mind which has the problem of knowing very often that it does not know or have all the answers. The thinking mind and knowing mind are not exactly separate in the way depicted above but have a much more fluid working arrangement. This is the frustration of thinking mind because it knows from some deep part of itself that it is limited to time and space and linear processes and so generally wont ask for help unless desperate. That is the arrogance and narrow mindedness of Ego.

The conscious thinking mind would like a bit of the pie and would like to have the knowing, creative depth and silent presence of what it regards as its deeper self but this is not easily available via thinking. Thinking mind can only think, that is its operative way and when no thinking is taking place then one becomes aware of the silence of the non-linear knowing mind, which is always present.

So here is the crux of the problem. The thinking mind using the 'I' word identifies with what it thinks is the 'real self' when it is in reality a small part of the total SELF. The total self includes the conscious and unconscious/knowing' mind. The problem is that the conscious mind cannot become the unconscious mind.

For whatever reason they have different functions, 'fields of operation', and ways of working. Thinking cannot become non-thinking or to put it another way, to enter into the non-thinking territory, thinking must slow down and even stop. In that moment the non-thinking mind takes over as it were. I have discussed this in different ways in other chapters as well.

How does this relate to the God story and the big question, does God/Great Mystery take part in healing?

This question has occupied much of my mind over the last 35 years. During this time I was engrossed in trying every tool and natural medicine coming my way. To my surprise a great many of them worked. In fact everything I tried seem to work in some people. The techniques I remained with for longer periods of time were just the ones that seemed more consistent in their results, were easier to fit into my practice and were more acceptable to more patients and my profession. These techniques also resonated with me and therefore felt right and required no effort. Nevertheless everything I tried seemed to work.

At one point I became so frustrated in trying to hone in on the practice and management protocols that worked the best that I decided that it was not the tools or medicines that made any real difference and that 'I' was the common factor in all these approaches and so perhaps all that was needed was 'myself' which included my approach, my hands and voice and the environment that patients came too.

To test this out I decided to do one simple thing. Firstly to stop using all the machines and tools I had available (low energy lasers, acupuncture needles, Bicom, Rife etc.) and just get the patients to lie on the bed facing downwards while I placed my hands on their back moving them downwards along the spine and along the limbs as if I was examining the patient.

I did this procedure for a few patients and then decided this was very boring and went back to doing what made me sing i.e. using the acupuncture needles and other tools which I loved using.

What I learnt from this experience is that while I still am not sure that the tools I used to support healing and even the remedies given to patients are the main vehicles to stimulate healing in the patient, there is a very real 'practitioner' aspect to the healing process and why the placebo response is so important and can vary from one practitioner to another even though they may be using the same drug or even doing surgery. In the chapter on the placebo response I noted that just cutting the skin and stitching without the full operation was enough to move people from a non functioning painful joint to full function despite the fact that no surgery apart from cutting the skin had actually been done to change the pathology.

Where does God fit into the story?

Who is present in the room with the doctor and his patient?

Two human bodies, yes for sure but what else is present. In the chapter on the 'greater anatomy' of the human being I wrote about the matter- energy- information- quantum space system and body- emotions- mind- consciousness system and that this is what constitutes the bigger human anatomy.

So in asking the question who is in the room besides the two bodies it becomes obvious that much more is going on than just a conversation which can be recorded. The HeartMath organisation have measured the electromagnetic recordings of the heart with very sensitive instruments discovered that it is possible to measure this recording almost one metre away from the body. This is a complex recording and what exactly is transferred when two people are sitting close enough for these recordings to entangle is unknown.

In reviewing my experience of working with patients and living life as a very aware individual over almost 40 years I have made the following deductions around health and healing:

- There is a vast hidden depth to reality that is not accessible to logical linear thinking mind or reductionistic science.

- That logical thinking mind can only think and that this thinking is conditioned by training, experience and the very limitations of sensory organs. The eyes only see a limited range of light frequencies and the ears only hear a limited range of sound. All our senses are limited and therefore the information we receive is filtered information and clearly not all that is available. Animals with difference sensory apparatus are able to see, hear, and feel etc. a different reality to that of humans.

- From this very limited information our thinking mind with its background of conditioning, training, education and experience constructs a limited view of reality. It is difficult to know how limited this viewpoint is because the rest of reality is unknown.

- We can enlarge our view of reality by using instruments that go beyond our own sensory apparatus. These instruments and tools include a range of biochemical investigation, x-rays, sonars and magnetic resonances. These extend our knowledge of reality beyond those of our senses but still remains within the realm of linear, reductionistic science.

- Any measuring apparatus however is still limited by the fact that it can only measure what it can measure and therefore has its own set of limitations and boundaries. The apparatus is still dependent on the human thinking mind in order to make sense of the report. The human thinking mind as indicated is itself limited to linear logical processes.

- Reality is not linear but functions in the round, holistically, creatively, purposefully and intelligently.

- Systems are everywhere and these systems especially living systems are open to the outer environment and connected to an inner environment. Systems cannot be broken apart without loosing their holistic integrity.

- The conscious thinking linear mind works in co-operation with a non-thinking, knowing, and non-linear mind.

- The thinking mind has created the 'scientific paradigm', which is the outer manifestation of its linear thinking processes, where everything functions in a linear way and for every effect there is a preceding cause. The thinking mind tries to maintain control of this narrow minded reality by excluding the 'subjective' and any experience that cannot be measured and seems 'mysterious'.

- Living systems are intelligent, have knowingness around their habitat, survival, food requirements and the balance of things. Without thinking they are able to survive, develop resistance to chemicals, which the human thinking minds create to kill them. Birds, bees, ants, bats all survive in colonies, which serve the whole and function in harmony. Thinking can marvel at this co-operation and recognizes the inherent cohesiveness of this life.

So there we have it. A strange reality indeed or should I say that the way we perceive reality is extremely limited. Bye reducing reality to only that which can be perceived by our senses, interpreted by our thinking mind and measured by our tools and instruments we may believe that we really know a great deal. I guess my point is that all that we know is still a limitation based on the narrowness of our senses, the tools we use to measure and the basic nature of the thinking mind, which cannot grasp a reality beyond thought.

We are dealing with complex systems and approaches and relying on objective experimentation, logical deduction and reductive thinking, will limit complexity to linear non-complex processes. The real world appears unlikely to conform to this kind of reality. Paul Cilliers, Professor in the Department of Philosophy and a world expert in 'complexity studies' makes the following statements in a short draft on 'The limits of understanding'.

"There is an inescapable normative dimension to all things complex. This implies that the claims we make about complex things are always provisional and limited. Such claims should thus be made with a certain humility.'

He points out that a great deal of work dealing with complex systems tends to revert to the traditional reductive way of explanation. This may be useful but the limitations of this approach in describing complex systems needs to be recognised. This understanding of the limits of science allows researchers perhaps to accept the importance of the 'art' of medicine.

Healing in the end is a strange mixture of science and art. The art is the confounding part of the process and in a way is a perturbation of the precise science that scientists examining living systems would really like to have. This is the downfall of pure science much to the frustration of medical scientists. Trying to separate the nuts and bolts of living systems in order to examine the nuts and bolts leaves out the 'organic and creative living quality'. One is now dealing with parts only and these don't exist in a living system which functions as a unified whole.

Can living systems be subjected to the kind science we are using today in medical research. I am not really sure that one can! Living systems are astonishingly complex and as indicated above, trying to reduce them to simple parts in order to examine them may be useful but if it denies the complexity and becomes a way of controlling or creating rigid protocols then medical science looses the creative edge and become dogmatic and narrow minded. This is not good science but scientism.

The individual is unique in every way. The underlying causes of ill health are unique to that person. The way the system as a whole responds to these causes is also unique so that the outcomes are not predictable, much to our frustration. Doctors and their patients may want clear answers but unfortunately this will never be possible. Complexity in living systems does not stand-alone but includes 'creativity' and 'wholeness' embedded in a universe that appears to be soaked in consciousness.

Medical science has I believe got stuck in its own initial success with antibiotics and not moved much from then, still exploring the next magic bullet to heal all disease. As Professor Kriel points out[2]: 'The real world is complex, plurivocal, richly textured with the potential for multiple significance. It has many meanings that require a plurality of ways of understanding. These meanings cannot be reduced to that of the physical sciences'. He has called for a broader understanding of 'science' that includes a better understanding of consciousness as well.

Fritjof Capra who has written extensively about the paradigm shift required in medicine has something similar to say.

'The Cartesian paradigm was based on the belief that scientific knowledge could achieve absolute and final certainty. In the new paradigm it is recognised that all concepts, theories and findings are limited and approximate. Science can never provide any complete and definitive understanding of reality'.

That too is a very powerful statement from a physicist. It seems that many physicists dealing with the complexity of modern science and what quantum science has added to this understanding are becoming more comfortable with the whole concept of 'uncertainty' lurking everywhere.

Modern medicine is still stuck in the old science, convinced that the magic bullet to treat disease will still be found using the tools of the old science. No one really talks any longer about the 'war against cancer' as if the battle will be won soon, and while scientists love to talk about breakthroughs and really exciting progress, not much has changed in the last decade.

Statistics may suggest that the medical profession is really doing quite well with cancer management but generally this is more about the increasing diagnosis of early cancers of the breast, prostate and thyroid. This however distorts the stats of cancer prognosis because it is becoming clear that many of these cancers don't spread, grow so slowly that people die with them and not from them spreading and may even spontaneously disappear. Chemotherapy is seriously toxic and it is not clear that the battle against cancer is anywhere close to being resolved.

2   Conversations 2.Aforum for the changing Health Paradigm. 2014

The same applies to all diseases. Real breakthroughs are hard to come by. This is not difficult to understand if one is clear about the nature of complexity and what it means for living systems. I suggest that the way of doing research in medicine needs to shift. There needs to be a deeper understanding that we are not dealing with 'parts' interacting with each other but interactive open creative systems that are following an intelligence and consciousness that is far beyond the limited logical thinking mind and self centered egoist understanding.

In searching for information on complexity on YouTube I came across this evangelical Christian show in which a number of people were talking about miracle cures that had happened to them. This included fibromyalgia, serious allergy problems including asthma and another person who had been blind for four years. All cured instantaneously and miraculously.

There are too many stories like this to dismiss all of them. I have personally had two miraculous spontaneous healing. Both involved back pain. One was upper back and the other lower back. In each case the pain was seriously debilitating and in both cases, which were years apart, sudden healing happened through my own efforts and desire to find a way out. I write more about these healings in the chapter on my personal story.

I am well aware of the power of the placebo, hypnosis and prayer and while these are generally dismissed as just 'mind over matter', one needs to ask exactly what do people mean by this statement. If you mean that the mind can make miracles happen, can heal the body from serious disease then that is a most important statement. The first article I ever wrote was in my final year of medical school and was a study of 'mind over matter'.

I guess I have always been fascinated by the possibilities of the power of the mind. What I realise now is that it is not the logical thinking left brain that seems involved in the miraculous but the right brain. So asking the left brain with its logical abilities and thinking in a linear way to try and understand its polar opposite which is the right creative non linear mind is just not going to happen.

This is the conflict we have also between the science and the art of medicine. Scientists try and confine their approach to logical linear science using the left brain without understanding that this is only one way of understanding living systems which don't really function in this way and that miraculous healing can 'break through' as it were to initiate a healing process.

As humans we operate with both left and right brains, with logic and intuition, with head and heart. As health professionals, depending on our personality types, we may approach patients from a purely logical framework or from a more heartfelt space.

Many practitioners manage to combine both approaches. Medical science however has chosen a much more left brain approach in which there is little space for miracles, intuition and the art of medicine even though those same medical scientists may be religious and even believe in the miracles of prayer, intuitive breakthroughs in their own understanding, and the complexity of personal relationships.

Scientists live dual lives. At home they may be all heart but when they pass through those doors of their workplace, they don their scientific hats and then forget that living systems are not machines which can be only understood by breaking apart, but are miraculous systems far beyond their ability to fully comprehend.

We certainly need to be careful about exaggerated claims for Natural approaches for cancer treatment for example and constantly pointing to the serious sided effects of chemotherapy without also pointing to the possibility that surgery, chemotherapy and radiation may be life saving to many people.

Nevertheless we do have a problem here. Much of the work around natural approaches to cancer and the results are anecdotal and generally include people that have already had surgery and some chemotherapy or radiation and a great deal of the results of conventional therapy are as indicated from people whose cancer may never have spread. So it is confusing and easier to talk about the statistics than what each person needs in order to have the best outcome.

Statistics can easily be manipulated depending on the outcome one wants leaving the poor patient in a predicament. Do you trust your doctor who generally has a very biased viewpoint, your Integrative doctor who has his or her own particular bias yet also understands the enormous complexity involved and that his experience is always going to be limited and may not apply to your particular case.

No one knows the Absolute Truth and Exactly what is Required in your case.

Like weather forcasting, there is an inherent spontaneity in nature that makes any prediction guesswork based on experience.

As Gary Player, a South African world champion golfer once said; 'The more I practice, the luckier I get.' In the end this is also true of medicine. Perhaps a scary truth for most of us to sit with, that is, in each case the outcome of management is always going to be a surprise. There is so much complexity at work, so many thousands upon thousands of processes, entangled together that any prediction is pure guesswork.

The more experience, the better the guesswork.

Karl Popper in his book The Logic of Scientific Discovery (1959) says the following:

'Science does not rest upon solid bedrock. The bold structure of its theories rises, as it were, above the swamp. It is like a building erected upon piles. The piles are driven down from above the swamp, but not down to any natural or 'given' base.'

Where does this leave the doctor and the patient and how to respond to this kind of information?

We all know that human beings are fallible, that we tend to find what is being looked for, that no one is really unbiased but is influenced by personal ambition, preconceptions, prejudices and a range of other pressures to get particular results.

Patients also want to hear certain outcomes that are positive and reflect their particular culture and view of the world. The result is that everyone is working pretty hard to maintain a level of order in their life and ideas of complexity, chaos, creativity, mystery and the Great Unknown does not always sit well with us.

Yet, the truth is that we are dealing with unpredictability, a great mystery that will not disappear, black holes that we know very little about and yet makes up much of the universe around us and scientific methods that have not resolved this dilemma but in recent times with the introduction of quantum science has only pointed even more to the great mystery around us. To top if off the greatest mystery of all may be the nature of consciousness itself. We know we are conscious and yet the very nature of consciousness deludes all our investigations.

Very recently I was telling my wife how nice it would be if I had the ability to see into the future or had some kind of psychic power and ability to heal. I was convinced that this ability would make me a better doctor and help in identifying management protocols that worked.

That night I had a dream. In the dream I was asked whether I really wanted to have the ability to see into the future. I was shown a young couple with their 3-year-old child and could see that the child would die within a few weeks and that nothing I did could heal it. I was also given to see the look of absolute horror in the face of the parents when I told them this prediction. I was then asked if I still wanted this predictive ability and could I take full responsibility for this gift. The alternative I was made aware of was to just trust that life would always be doing its best provided I was doing my best to respond to the situation.

I decided that I did not need that gift and that I was quite prepared to hand it over to a much Greater Intelligence of which my 'non thinking' mind seems to be part of.

So there we have it.

It seems to me that I have come to understand that the 'thinking mind' would love to be in control of outcome but that this is actually arrogant and an ego driven idea of control. Just letting go outcomes and recognising that there is much more at work here, that complexity reigns supreme, that what we don't know and may never know because of complexity and the thinking mind's narrow field of expertise has been a major revelation and allowed me to relax in my work as healer.

I do want people to get healed and feel joyful and I will continue to try to achieve this outcome but deep within there is another joy of just allowing life to move its own creative way knowing that there is another intelligence at work. If anyone want to call this intelligence God then that is really okay. I personally prefer to use the word 'Great Mystery' which reminds me of the nature of the mystery in life, the complexity present everywhere and the nature of healer as both artist and scientist together.

Chapter 22

He is one of South Africa's top medical scientists, recognised throughout the world for his contribution to sports medicine and honoured many times by international bodies for his research. He has challenged some common and old paradigms in sports medicine and nutritional medicine and performed the research to prove the correctness of his views. He has received some of the top awards that South Africa has to offer. In 2002, he was awarded the International Cannes Grand Prix Award for research in Medicine and yet today he has had to defend himself in front of colleagues because of his outspoken views on the standard version of the diet reccomended by the medical establishment and which clearly has not led to better health but an epidemic of obesity and diabetes. An invitation to attend a medical congress has been withdrawn and colleagues have turned against him and closed ranks around their dietary advice despite its obvious failure.

The New Emerging Medicine

As one approaches the end of this book a pattern begins to emerge which can give some indication of what the new medicine will possibly look like. Paradigm shifts occur throughout the ages. A paradigm is defined as a 'model' or 'pattern' and a paradigm shift suggests a change in the model and the understanding one had before. Some major paradigm shifts have occurred over the centuries but perhaps the most significant one that interests us was the shift from the Middle Ages to Modern times.

In Chapters 2 and 3 we discussed the history of thought and the movement from magical thinking to scientific reductionistic mathematical approaches to life. This latter approach focused on material reality, lawfulness, rationality and logic pushing magic, intuition, relationship with nature and the cosmos into the background. In the latter approach the universe was seen to be alive; angels, spirits, gods, animals communicated with humans who established a hierarchy, symbolic stories and organised metaphors to understand the world as they perceived it.

But this all changed very dramatically between 1600 and 1700, changing the medieval into the modern era as we recognize it today. The work of scientists and the stories and metaphors they used to explain the world based on their discoveries changed our view of reality in a most profound way.

We have all had the experience of looking at a painting and thinking how uninteresting it looked until the artist came along and explained what motivated him to paint what he did and what each stroke represented. Suddenly the painting takes on another whole dimension and one sees far beyond that which initially appeared to be there and yet it is the same painting. As more and more people agree with the artist the painting which initially may have disinterested everyone takes on an aura of something quite special and even mind expanding.

Magical experienced based approach to life vs a rational scientific thinking approach.

So it is with paradigm shifts. A new description of the world captures the imagination of everyone, and in the case of the change to the modern era it claimed to be based on facts rather than experience, subjectivity and magic. What needs to be clear however is that very often what appear to be facts are only part of the picture and therefore not completely true and that descriptions of reality may be exactly that, only descriptions or metaphors which we use to organize facts and therefore not much different to any other description of the world, only perhaps more effective for what is required at that time.

Let me explain because this is quite important. Reality is not that easy to capture. Only look around the world and see how everywhere there are a different points of view regarding reality.

Reality is a moving target!

This happens to apply also to scientists despite the fact that they claim to deal only with objectivity and the measured world. The eyes can only see and not hear. The same limitation applies to any investigating tool. They are devices and like the eye or any sensory organ give a view of reality which is limited by the scope of the device and therefore not a view of reality but only what the machine can measure.

It turns out that the world of matter and reality is much more complex than initially envisioned. As scientists delve more and more into the natural world and investigate biological systems, it begins to appear that the laws of science as applied to machines do not work for living and even non living systems. Here is the crux of the next paradigm shift.

Do the scientific laws which apply to machines also apply to living systems?

The Newtonian materialistic world does seem to apply to the machine world created by scientists and we have been living a machine reality. The metaphors of scientist have re-inforced this reality and many people believe that they are bodies walking around that have learned to think and that their bodies work in a clearly defined way, just much more complicated than any sophisticated machine. They believe also that the universe around them follows mathematical laws and from the time of the big bang expanded according to these clearly defined laws. Scientist have created machine metaphors based on their developing understanding as they organize facts and observations into a tapestry which makes sense to them.

But suddenly all this is changing and the tapestry of science is starting to look frayed and even unreal as frontier scientist begin to point out exceptions which don't fit in and measurements which don't support the conventional reality. The tapestry began to shift slowly at first but then with such increasing speed that many scientists and reality seekers started recognising a major paradigm movement in the. The more conventional scientists holding on to the old paradigm are beginning to look a little like the 'flat earth' society members who believed the world was flat even after the first ship had sailed to the edge and found no edge.

New facts emerging which don't fit neatly into the conventional models developed by scientists over the last century.

The shift has emerged because new facts can no longer be fitted into the present understanding and these facts are giving another view of reality. Of special interest is that scientists are beginning to connect ancient knowledge of the world with many of these new scientific discoveries. These are really exciting times as we begin to redefine our present reality and begin to recognise the limited viewpoint we have been living with. It seems that reality is not a fixed structure but is a constant moving tapestry of changing colours, textures and tones.

The terminology of the new science and the new paradigm is of special interest to us as we begin to look in particular how it affects our view of medicine and what the new medicine will look like. The change won't be easy. Human beings like to believe that they have a priority on their particular viewpoint, which is based on facts and their experience and therefore must be more right that, their neighbour.

We kill, excommunicate, banish, ban, jail and even torture those whose viewpoint differs from our own. Good scientists with alternative viewpoints even when backed by good reseach find themselves pretty lonely, invitations to conferences no longer come their way and research grants dry up very quickly .

Paradigm shifts suggest that major changes in thought about reality can take place and should make us very wary of trying to limit our view of reality. Our view of reality is always only a view and nothing more. As we are plunged into the new world there is going to be great confusion and stress for those that refuse to budge from their chosen point of view.

The new science has developed a terminology that reflects a reality that is shifting and dynamic and yet has order and even mathematical precision. I have listed below some of the terminology used to describe this new viewpoint.

- Systems
- Webs
- Non-linear dynamics
- Fields of force
- Energy
- Informational systems
- Connectiveness, coupling, bonding
- Holism
- Patterns
- Probability dynamics
- Relationships
- Sacred geometry
- Meaning
- Self-organisation
- Turbulence

- Order and Chaos

- Spirit in science and science of spirit

- Intuition

- Experience

- Microcosm and macrocosm

- Non-locality (the great physics riddle)

- Upward causation and downward causation.

- Complexity

- Consciousness

Words such as intuition and experience may sound a little corny when applied to 'science' but some of the best scientists are beginning to recognize that the observer and what is observed cannot be separated and are increasingly looking at the role of consciousness in the scientific process. As we move to define the new medicine some of the above metaphors will begin to look quite attractive but let us start at a more basic level and at one of the defining themes of the new medicine, which really does separate it from the conventional viewpoint.

Improving health vs treating disease

Conventional medicine seems to be stuck in a paradigm in which the treatment of disease has become a priority. The disease is the most physical aspect of the problem and therefore most easily identified, localised and then treated. Not surprising therefore that doctors find it easier to concentrate their attention on this aspect of the ill health .

The fascination with the disease and pathology has tended to overshadow the underlying functional disturbances which precede the disease and the causes which precede the dysfunction. The complexity and time involved in searching for causes has also led to the focus on the disease and finding drugs to alleviate the symptoms. Unless of course the cause seems obvious, as in infections when antibiotics are used to treat the problem.

As indicated in previous chapters even here the cause is not so obvious when one penetrates more deeply into the situation. Bacteria of themselves cannot cause a problem unless the immune system is unable to prevent this from happening and the immune system is disturbed and rendered weak by multiple factors which include toxins, lack of supportive nutrients, poor sleep etc. Suddenly the underlying cause is no longer straight forward.

Using powerful drugs to control the symptoms of the disease becomes a simple approach to getting a quick result without having to deal with the complexity of the situation. The drugs which are used have significant effects and side effects on the physiological processes in the body which will bring up the question of benefits vs harm. In other words are the benefits of the symptomatic improvement of the disease worth the harm that may arise from long term use over years.

Benefits of drugs vs risks! Who knows the truth?

Most research is directed and financed by pharmaceutical companies so that the focus on the disease remains very central to all medical management .At the same time biochemists(the majority working for or being paid by pharmaceutical companies) continue to search for biochemical answers to treating the disease rather than healing the person.

Treating the disease vs healing the person.

In the New Medicine there is the recognition that healing is a natural process taking place constantly in the body. At the end of the day we are all exhausted, have difficulty in concentration have little motivation and yet in the morning one wakes up refreshed, full of energy and ready to go again.

No drug or other medicine is necessary for this to happen, it is a natural process in which the body is able to renew and refresh itself and bring back more health than the evening before. Despite this very profound difference in experience between the way we feel on going to bed and waking up in the morning there is little physiological changes to explain this remarkable difference.

The difference between being beat up and exhausted at the end of the day and alive and ready to go in the morning is so extraordinary that one should be surprised to learn that very little research is going on in this area. A natural sleep can do for the body what no medication can do. Sleep research for example has shown that 'short sleepers' (5 hours/night) have much less insulin sensitivity than 'normal sleepers' (8 hours /night). A decrease in insulin sensitivity leads over time to diabetes 2. A decrease in sleep by 1.5 hours reduces peformance by 32% and just by correcting sleep problems, ADD and ADHD can dissapear.

Practitioners of the new medicine have a great respect for drugs and the powerful and effective surgical techniques now available but they have an equal respect and fascination for the body systems own healing potential. They also understand that when the healing processes in the body become inefficient and ineffective then the seeds of ill health are sown.

The new medicine will therefore combine these two powerful themes:

- Improve Health

- Treat the disease where appropriate without weakening health if possible.

The new medicine will also begin to reflect the 'new science'.

Quantum mechanics and systems theory as indicated throughout this book had a profound effect on the thinking of Integrative doctors but little influence on the medicine practised by most doctors today. As indicated in other chapters modern medicine is still following a reductionistic linear paradigm in which there is a preceding cause for all ill health, that the body is made up of parts and that treating disease requires one to find the pathway of that ill health and then produce a drug that interferes with that pathway.

The recognition of multiple causes also suggests that the effects of multiple causes will also tend to be directed in a number of directions so that one may end up with multiple areas of the system involved.

Multiple causes - - - > Many effects - - - > Disease

The New Medicine recognizes this complexity. Quantum mechanics has already identified this complexity in Chaos theory and the butterfly effect. Chaos theory does not mean that everything is chaotic but rather than systems are so complex that it is difficult to know exactly what is going on, yet there does seem to be an underlying order.

Weather is a good example. With all the tools at our disposal we can only guess what the weather will be like in a few days' time. It seems chaotic yet there is some underlying order in the flow of the seasons and the movement of weather conditions. The butterfly effect indicates that a butterfly flapping it wings in New York could cause a storm in San Francisco i.e. small input can have very profound effects.

A small thought can cause my hand to go up. An emotion which cannot be measured can cause turmoil in the physiological processes of the body. It is clear to many scientists now that when information or energy enters into a dynamic creative and complex system there is no way to predict what will emerge.

It is also clear that physiological explanations as described in classic text books of physiology are only explanations based on ideal and linear thinking processes. If physiological processes were linear in reality i.e. one effect leading to another effect as it is in your motor car or other mechanical machine then life would not be able to exist. Living systems are much too complex for this to be true with billions of processes happening in every moment of time and moving in many different directions almost instantaneously.

Instead the new science and the terminology developed gives us metaphors to begin to understand how complex systems do work. The biological system is a web of activity in which each apparent part is connected to every other part and responds immediately to any change anywhere in the system.

Energy and information flows throughout the system at lightening speeds creating patterns of activity, which maintain balance and harmony. In seems that there is order and this order has been known to the ancients who saw in the shells on the beach, in the tigers stripes, in the patterns of the stars, in the way birds flew in formation, in the symmetry of structure in flowers and species specificity, an order which is now referred to as sacred geometry. This same sacred geometry patterns were used to build the temples, houses and even cities in ancient times.

Biological living systems are webs of activity interacting in multiple complex ways.

And yet…and yet at the same time the ancients recognised and were awed at the creativity in nature and the world around them. Change seemed to move hand in hand with order and it was this changing aspect of life that created fear and drew men and women together to protect themselves from natures capriciousness.

It was the wise men and wise women of the times that understood this relationship and were able to guide and advise.

The old Newtonian science discovered the order; the new science is infatuated with the changing creative side. The new medicine at last recognizes that the human being as a system does not function like a machine. That there is order within change and change within order. Much more complex than the weather, more creative than sophisticated computers and constantly confounding the predictions of biochemists.

What is the response of Integrative practitioners to this information?

Integrative practitioners recognize this complexity:-

- recognize that there are no single causes.

- that the effects may spread out over the body causing multiple symptoms and signs.

- that these symptoms and signs reflect an underlying diffuse process which is complex and has numerous points of origin and endpoints.

- that the system functions as one piece and not as separate parts.

- that there is an underlying intelligence in the system which needs to be respected as it is always trying to heal and maintain harmony.

How does this translate into a functional approach to health and disease? Integrative practitioners tend not to treat ill health in isolation.There is illness and there is health. Illness is still the best the system can do under the circumstances. It is not 'wrong' but the best effort the system can do in order to maintain balance. Trying to 'correct the illness' by throwing in chemical drugs which intefere with function will only place more stress on the system. While symptomatic help is occassionally the right thing to do , it does come at a cost of increasing strain on the systems intelligence to maintain balance.

The whole system body/emotions/mind is involved and needs to be taken into account in the management of ill health. Thus the patient with headaches, menstrual bleeding and sleep disturbance does not have 3 different conditions requiring 3 separate drugs and possible 3 different specialists to investigate the problem but a practitioner who can see the whole picture.

The whole system is always involved in any 'disease'. Nothing happens in isolation.

The headache, menstrual bleeding and sleep disturbance are only the outer expression of a disturbance of function within the system which for what ever reason cannot be corrected by the intelligence within the system. There cannot possible be separate conditions in a system, which is intelligent and must have immediate access to all that is happening throughout its multilevel structure.

Thoughts, emotions, temperature changes, digestion, breathing patterns, level of physical activity all will cause physiological changes which must be adjusted and corrected in order to maintain the very fine balance of pH and temperature controls and other homeostatic mechanisms necessary for good health.

When the system starts to break down it does not suggest that chaos now is dominant. Even in a very ill person the remarkable degree of health still present is quite astonishing. Even days before a patient dies digestion, oxygen consumption and healing of wounds may still be occurring relatively normally. All this suggests a highly sophisticated and intelligent system which is generally in control .If there is ill health the whole system tries to maintain function and will do so despite enormous odds.

The whole system is always trying its best to maintain aliveness and balance. It will always be doing the best it can do to maintain homeostasis. Even the dying process is controlled by the body's systems and is the best it can do under the circumstances. Anything we as doctors do should support this intelligence. Poor diet, stress and the wrongful use of natural products and drugs will intefere with the complexity of responses required to maintain health..

Integrative practitioners are aware that their function is primary to support the intelligence of the system maintain optimum function and secondly to remove any blocks to healing.

Maintenance of Optimum Function Removes Blocks to Healing

We are now ready to define the New Medicine which perhaps can be best described as Integrative Medicine.

It has the following tenets:

- An expansion from reductionism to Holism and yet recognising the value of examining parts.

- The recognition that the human being is a system functioning as one piece rather than parts linked together.

- A quantum mechanical understanding, which does not exclude the value of Newtonian physics.

- An expansion from a biochemical understanding to include a bio-energetic viewpoint.

- An enlargement even of this viewpoint to include information

Information<--->Energy<----->Matter

- The inclusion of a psycho-spiritual understanding within the mind-body connection to include 'meaning' and the 'journey of life' for example.

- Investigations to include the functional integrity of the system.

- That the system as a whole is always maintaining the best balance it can. Ill health and disease still fall within the system's domain and is the best the system can do. Homeostasis or balance will still be present in the system despite the ill health or disease.

Ill health is not 'wrong' but the best the body can do under the circumstances.

Almost all investigations such as X rays, MRIs, biopsies, urine and blood measurements, sonars etc. are looking at the body parts as a section frozen in time. Non-conventional functional tests include Dark Field Microscopy in which a drop of blood is examined without being stained and fixed and allows one to assess the movement and shape of cells within the blood in real time.

The central dogma of the Integrative method is the deepening understanding that the whole system is involved in trying to maintain harmony and balance despite the toxins in the environment, the up and down of emotional stress, the underlying nutritional deficiencies and all the other factors mentioned in the chapter on causes.

The management protocol then is hinged on helping the system return back to better harmony with less stress on the system . As this happens the symptoms and signs will slowly dissapear and if the diseased part of the body can return to better function then even that will dissapear or become much less of a problem.

From the above perspective the modern medical approach seems rather strange. Using chemical drugs which are powerful enough to block physiological processes will obviously increase the stress in the system. The system as indicated is always doing the best it can do. What it needs is support to physiology and not blocks. Those support streams include:

- Serious life style changes as discussed

- Removing blocks and interfering factors. These include all pollutants and drugs if possible.

- Stress reduction

- Optimising nutritional needs

With these simple steps the system can begin its healing proces. It really knows what to do.

Health and healing is its basic function.

The living system knows how to heal itself. Support the system.

All this should be obvious and be the very first step in management of ill health, nevertheless the vast majority of doctors are not taught how to support health but to treat the disease with powerful chemicals. The lay public have better insight into the first step of management and are often doing some of this already by the time they visit their doctor. Not much point in talking to their doctor about lifestyle management.

The doctor is already pulling out the prescription pad to write down a few drugs required to help the symptoms. Integrative doctors on the other hand begin right here at lifestyle management helping the person make diet choices, exercise motivation and stress management. If the Integrative practitioner pulls out the prescription pad then it is usually to write down some nutritional product which will support health rather than treat symptoms.

Practitioners of Integrative Medicine are well trained in both the Art and Science of medicine and recognize the value of science while at the same time not denigrating experience.

Another really important aspect of the Integrative method concerns the practitioner. Not much point in telling people what to do if you don't do it yourself.

"Healer know thyself" and be an example of health promotion.

'Healer know thyself' was written above the entrance of the Hippocrates School of medicine on the Greek island of Kos thousands of years ago. Theories can be learnt but if you have not walked the path then the theory will come without compassion, humility and the knowingness that arises from having walked the path and learnt how unique it is for each individual. Theories are maps but not the territory. Practitioners of Integrative medicine should also have participated in some form of self analysis and psychotherapy in order to be fully present, compassionate and open to dialogue with their patient..

It is really difficult to move away from the idea that by diving deeper and deeper into the mechanism that drive systems we will find out how they actually function. This idea is so deeply imbedded into our psyche that even as children we will break our toys to find the rattle within.

Once the toy is broken and the source of the sound discovered then the toy is now useless and is thrown away in disgust. There is something quite fascinating however in the same discovery as an adult. Despite the fact that the toy is destroyed in breaking it apart, there is still the deep satisfaction in at least discovering something quite special about the way things function.

What have we gained in this process and what have we lost? We have gained some insight into the structure but not about its functional integrity. To understand about structure is one thing but to understand about function is another. I often refer to this problem as the difference between the map and the territory. By breaking the system into parts we build up maps that allow others to reproduce those structures.

The map has little to really say about function and when we are dealing with living systems then this is vital. A examination of the body of a dead person can tell us very little about that person apart from the anatomy and will not even help us to know much of the functional integerity of that body. Human beings as indicated in the chapter on 'the larger anatomy' are an amazing complex system, unique and creative in many ways.

The Integrative Holistic Systems based approach to medicine recognises this difference and takes care to keep in mind that while reducing the human being to anatomy and parts practitioners much also remember to step back to see the whole and the way that unique being is functioning.

I can now summerize some of the important 'pillars' of the new Medicine emerging:

- The human being is a system in which all the parts are seeminglessly integrated to function as a whole.

- The greater anatomy; matter-energy-information- quantum space and Body– emotions- mind-consciousness.

- The recognition that there are no single causes for any illness i.e. all illnesses are multicausal.

- An emphasis on supporting health rather than treating disease

- Moving dysfunction back to function i.e. improving the functional integrity of the system.

- Holism

- Biochemical individuality i.e. each person is unique right down the line from anatomy to physiology, to genetic profiles and probably into the energy streams.

- The very serious link between consciousness and the way the body functions i.e. mind-body are not two separate parts joined together, they are much more like the top and bottom of a pencil. There is no top without a bottom and no bottom without a top. One could say that the one end is the active doing end and the other is the storage or nourishing end. The one end is the masculine active end and the other the feminine nourishing and supporting end.

- Joins the Art and Science of medicine into a single flowing process i.e. making a diagnosis from the blood tests only without recognising the unique whole person who has come for the consultation is not Integrative medicine but the old system. This does require a longer consultation without a focus only on 'making a diagnosis of disease'.

These are exciting times. Controversy in medicine is healthy and part of a progressive medical science provided of course that there is an open minded attitude to viewpoints that don't fit into the conventional paradigm. There are enormous pressures not to change the conventional paradigm with its focus on disease and the use of drugs and to label anyone with contrary viewpoints as charletans, too controversial and enemies of good scientific medicine.

'The crisis of our time isn't just a crisis of a single leader, organization, country, or conflict. The crisis of our time reveals the dying of an old social structure and way of thinking, an old way of institutionalising and enacting collective social forms.'[1]

'Science needs to be performed with the mind of wisdom.'[2]

'I am convinced that the sciences are being held back by assumptions that have hardened into dogmas, maintained by powerful taboos. These beliefs protect the citadel of established science, but act as barriers against open-minded thinking.'[3]

1   Scharmer C Otto. Theory U. BK publishers. 2009.p 2
2   Eleanor Rosch. University of California.
3   Rupert Sheldrake. The Science Delusion. Coronet 2012.page 12.

Chapter 23

My Personal Journey

My journey in medicine has followed a time line spanning over 55 years, from a very conventional medical training, specializing in gastrointestinal disorders, abandoning medicine for a period of 5years and then eventually returning to a medical practice when at the age of 38 years with the birth of our first child I realised that the practice of medicine was probably the best way for me to make a living in order to support a family.

I abandoned medicine while specialising in gastro- enterology in Miami, Florida. I had gone to America because I believed that in America one could live ones dream and it was so. It took me about 9 months to realise that despite living my dream I was still unhappy.

I had my dream car, a boat, a pretty good income with a good future already in place but that feeling that something was not quite right kept bugging me. Despite everything I had I remain discontented. Perhaps I thought I had made a mistake in becoming a doctor.

My special research involving pancreatic enzymes was boring, writing papers just to get grants and be somebody important in medicine did not excite me and even working with sick people in the hospital setting was uninteresting. At this point in my career I knew nothing about natural medicine or alternative medicine approaches and yet I was disillusioned with the conventional model and its focus on disease and the use of drugs to treat symptoms.

One early Sunday morning I woke up after a party at the house of a friend and we decided to play with a Frisbee in the street below before everyone woke up and the streets were still clear and quiet. It was my friend, an associated professor of pharmacology who shouted at me while we were running and playing that we should give up our jobs and find an island near Miami and move there to live our lives. He felt that we were intelligent enough to make a living anywhere and that working the way we did really sucked.

This was the first time such a thought had entered my mind but it seemed to resonate with some deep urge in my heart to find something more meaningful in my life that I did not at that time quite clearly understand..

The next day I walked into my boss's office and told him I was leaving medicine and would not return. He looked at me is disbelief. The laboratory and assistant were ready to go, I had really good opportunities and had just returned from visiting various labs around the USA and now was preparing to leave all this behind. It made no sense to him.

Giving up medicine and becoming an artist

My girlfriend at the time decided to leave her job as well which helped my decision and I moved into her house in order to save money. For the next few months we became artists. She painted and I did sculpture mainly from wood.

They were good times but no money was coming in and we were beginning to get worried.

One day while sitting rather glumly together wondering how to make a living a man walked in whom we had just met the previous day.

'So what's your problem?' he said, looking at our glum faces.

'Not making money from our art.' we said.

'Europe is the place to go for artists.' he said.

The governments in Europe, especially Holland, support the artists and commission them to work. What a great idea it seemed but we had cars, boats and other evidence of material wealth. So how much do you think it is worth he asked? Out came a cheque book and this stranger wrote out a cheque for the amount we believed all our possessions were worth. No questions asked and he disappeared.

Ten days later we were on our way to Europe, landing in Luxembourg and picking up our Volkswagen Kombi that we had bought and arranged to be at the airport when we arrived.

I looked at my girlfriend and said, so where do we go from here? It was decided to drive up to the northern part of Germany to the factory, which made the VW Kombis. We wanted to buy a box which fitted on the roof to carry our luggage items that we brought with us from the USA.

When we arrived at the factory we discovered a very large campsite filled with hippies and their VW Kombis waiting to be fitted out or fixed. We spent a couple of weeks in that campsite making friends and finding out where people travelled and how they lived travelling around Europe.

Hippie days

So it was that for the next three years we travelled in our VW Kombi going south to Spain or Greece in winter months and north mainly to Germany and Holland during the summer. These were interesting times. In retrospect I realise that these years were all about letting go of my conditioning around who I was and what I wanted to do with my life. Here I was living from day to day, with very little money, no permanent home, far from family, no permanent job, and just the stuff we could fit into the kombi which included at times two bicycles and a cat.

We were part of the hippie stream moving across Europe. It was the best of times from 1971 to about 1973. There was little crime within the community we travelled with, marijuana was freely available but hard drugs were not a major issue.

There was a great deal of sharing space, good music and talk of freedom, love and art. It was during these travels that I heard for the first time of spiritual talk; gurus in India, meditation, LSD and other hallucinogens and seeking one's authentic self or spirit.

I continued however to struggle with myself. It seemed to me that I should be happier than I was and that the promise of meditation, enlightenment, inner peace, astral travelling, past lives, ecstatic experiences that I kept reading about should also be part of my own life.

Meeting my Guru and teacher

So it was that in 1974 while on a visit to a friend in Amsterdam that I met my first Indian Guru, Dr. Kaushik. He was a medical doctor by profession, practicing in a small village in India. By chance a single Italian spiritual seeker was stuck in the little village Dr. Kaushik lived in because of a train breakdown and was taken to the home of the only English speaker in the village.

Dr. Kaushik apparently greeted him as if he was waiting for him to arrive. Within months, this Italian hippie had brought other travellers to the village until the people of the village asked the doctor to stop seeing these foreigners or leave with them. They were disturbed by so many foreigners walking around stoned from weed and felt the quiet life of their small village had changed since the invasion of these young people.

Dr. Kaushik left with his followers to a house he owned in the old city of Delhi and very soon this house became a haven for many westerners seeking spiritual teaching.

I can still remember the first question I asked Dr. Kaushik sitting on the floor of my friend's Amsterdam house.

I had been to a nightclub the night before and noted that there seemed to be two separate realities, the one reality with my eyes open and the other with my eyes closed.

'Which reality is the real one?' I asked him. His answer was that there was only one reality and that my mind was separating two aspects of the one reality. I think it took me many years to really understand that answer but at the time it struck me as a very wise answer and left me with the desire to see more of this man.

He invited us to visit him in Delhi if we were going in that direction. I had mentioned to him that we were planning to visit Sri Lanka and would be fairly close therefore to India. It was not our plan to visit India especially as it was almost impossible for a South African to obtain a visa to India. India and many other countries had stopped issuing visas to anyone from apartheid South Africa.

A few weeks later we gave our VW Kombi to a friend in Amsterdam to look after and left for Sri Lanka, which still welcomed South African citizens. Colombo is the capital city of Sri Lanka which at that time had just gained its independence from Britain but still retained all the Colonial trappings including grand buildings, good roads, English spoken everywhere, beautiful 'tea rooms' with doormen and butlers in uniform.

The downside was the over friendliness of the local people who seemed determined to practise their English on us. Everywhere we went we seemed to be followed by someone asking 'Where are you going?', 'Where do you come from?' or 'What is your name?' We soon learnt that most young travellers had gone down to the village of Hikkado on the coast. It was also a favorite place for the wealthy with grand hotels and famous coral reefs. That would be our destination we decided. The bus journey was about two hours and we had just emerged from the bus when we were accosted by a very well spoken 'gentleman' who offered us a room right on the edge of the beach.

This was off-season and the offer for board and breakfast was extremely cheap. In fact Sri Lanka turned out to be a really cheap haven for us with one dollar enough almost to feed us the whole day.

So it was that we spent the next year on the island of Sri Lanka. The island is tropical with coconut trees, Breadfruit trees and banana's growing pretty wild everywhere. The coral reef at that time was still unspoiled and it was possible to walk waist deep and see the most remarkable display of coral and coloured fishes of all sizes.

This really was paradise with great weather, brilliant sea temperature and sea life, long beaches with soft white sand, very friendly people, good fresh fish and an abundance of fruit and vegetables.

Despite all this I was surprised to discover after about 8 months that the same unhappiness that had followed me everywhere also began to raise its head even here. It is difficult to say exactly what it was. It did not feel like boredom because after years of travelling I had settled into living from moment to moment, with no responsibility. Our small income was more than sufficient in Sri Lanka.

We read, swam, walked, cooked great meals, painted and sat around having great conversations with the numerous young people passing along the hippie route from Tibet, through India to Sri Lanka. Many of these young people were buying gems in Sri Lanka to take back to their homes to sell.

The unhappiness I felt I realised was nothing to do with the place I was living in or my companion but clearly had to do with my own unhappiness with self. The books I was reading at the time were mainly about Buddhism, meditation, self-knowledge, spiritual growth and discovering more of the inner journey. I realised then that I would have to leave this island paradise and visit Dr Kaushik in India.

My first attempt to get a visa to visit India failed, as I was South African so I sent a telegram to Dr Kaushik in Delhi. Days later I received an answer telegram to return to the visa office and say that I was visiting my spiritual master and guide. My second application for a visa worked like magic, which convinced me of the special 'powers' of this guru teacher. It was much later that I discovered that one of his 'pupils' was also the minister of Health. My partner was Canadian and had no problem with her visa application.

Travelling to India

A few weeks later we were in Delhi and travelled to the old part of the city where Dr Kaushik lived in a small two room cottage. He slept in the one room with his helper and in the next room we slept with all the 'spiritual seekers'. As the oldest couple we were given a space under the staircase where there was a little more privacy. The rest of the room was filled with about 22 other young men and women. Most were Americans and had been living with the doctor for some months already.

There was a daily routine. An early morning walk, meditation in the local park, satsang (conversation) with the doctor in his small room and then lunch. After lunch we were free to visit the local teashop, walk in the park and chat or perhaps take a ride into the city of Delhi and visit some of the tourist sites.

There was one particular place I wanted to visit before leaving India and that was the Taj Mahal. This is one of the Seven Wonders of the World and I did not think that I would be visiting India again.

When I approached the doctor and asked for the day off to visit the Taj Mahal, he wanted to know why. When I told him that perhaps I would not be able to visit India again and so this was my one chance, he just laughed at me and said that this was a really poor reason for visiting. I clearly needed to find a much more spiritual reason for visiting and so a few day later I asked again and this time said that I understood that the Taj Mahal would shift me spiritually just by walking around it. The doctor laughed again, perhaps a little louder and told me again that my reasons were really not good enough.

So it was that week after week I would return to him with another reason for visiting and each time he would laugh louder and tell me to go back inside and think about it.

Weeks went by, even months, and it was almost time to leave. I was sitting in the park one morning, watching monkeys play in the trees and canaries flying from tree to tree, feeling somewhat deflated by not being able to find a reason to visit the Taj when very suddenly I had the following insight; 'the Taj Mahal that you are seeking to visit is not outside you but inside. Seek the temple within'.

That answer was so clear that I never again tried to visit the Taj Mahal and left India feeling as if that single moment had been all the teaching I needed from the Doctor.

The Taj Mahal you seek is within and not outside you.

Seeking within and no longer expecting answers in the 'outer world' became my real journey and mantra and in a way has continued to be my journey to this day.

The doctor had been invited to Europe and we decided to follow him and pick up our VW kombi from our friend who had been looking after it. He was returning to America so the timing again could not have been better.

We travelled with the doctor and a group of his students through Italy, Germany and then back to Amsterdam. In each country the reception was different. The Italians were more interested in just sitting with the doctor and sharing space with him. Their devotion and love was really special.

The Germans on the other hand wanted to debate spirituality and spend hours in conversation. The Dutch were a little bit of both with a deep respect for the wisdom of the man.

While travelling in Europe an invitation arrived for the doctor to visit America and because we had nothing else to do we decided to follow him to America. This would also give my partner and me time to visit her family in Canada. Our VW kombi was loaded onto a cargo ship and off it went to America while we flew into New York City to await its arrival and eventually join the doctor and friends somewhere in America.

Back to America

We travelled with the doctor for some months again. This time is rather vague in my mind. There were lots of deep discussions and really great venues but I can't remember any special revelations or insight. I continued struggling with my own stuff and emotional reactions, never quite feeling that I had discovered any greater truths that shifted me into another dimension of self. It felt that I had perhaps come to the end of my journey with the doctor and that it was time to move on.

Visiting family in Canada

We decided to visit my partner's family in Calgary and so we said goodbye to the doctor and all his students and our friends and off we went again in our VW Kombi to Calgary. It was summer in Canada everything was green, nevertheless Calgary was not an attractive city for someone coming from South Africa especially Cape Town and when Liz, my partner fell pregnant we decided that we should first get married in Calgary and then return to South Africa in order to bring up our children there. Of course we took our VW Kombi back with us to Cape Town.

Returning home

Six years after leaving South Africa I returned home. It had been an amazing journey. Perhaps the most important lessons had been letting go a great deal of my conditioning around money, place, religion and even family. I had come to realise that these were all trappings holding me in bondage; that I had tended to hold onto these ideas because they were a kind of security.

Money, religion and family all created a cushion, support and buffer from the crazy and even dangerous world out there. Letting all that go was both scary and exhilarating. Letting go of my needs to be secure threw me into the unknown but eventually helped me to discover an inner source of knowingness, trust and richness that would never have happened if it was not for my travelling and meeting Dr Kaushik. He had turned me to some deeper part of myself where I discovered a sense of freedom, wisdom and even love that had little to do with outward things.

I returned back to South Africa in 1976 and discovered that there was some money still left for me from my father's will. We were determined to bring up our children on a smallholding in the country and eventually found the perfect place above the town of Stellenbosch in the valley of Banhoek. It was about 1.4 hectares with a large house about 100 years old.

There were fruit trees and enough space to grow vegetables and even have a few animals. At this point in time I was still not thinking about returning to medicine and wondered whether growing organic vegetables and fruit could earn me a living. It did not take long to realise that this would not work. I was not a farmer at heart and the income would be pretty small; .nor did I have the capital to buy what I needed. Our first child, Joseph had arrived about five months after our return to South Africa.

About one year after arriving back in South Africa, there was a telephone call from a lady who had been the matron when I was still working in the local Cape Town hospital. She had heard of my return, was visiting Stellenbosch and wondered if she could come and visit together with a friend of hers.

This friend was an older lady, a homeopath who also turned out to be a spiritual teacher. During our afternoon conversation, she listened very carefully to my journey around parts of the world and my concern about making a living as a farmer.

'Well,' she said, 'how about returning back to medicine? You have trained for this and that can't be accidental or a mistake.' I guess I knew that all along and just needed someone to tell me that.

Starting a private practice in medicine

The decision to return back to the practice of medicine was not made lightly. I was out of touch, not really that interested in treating people with drugs and not knowing very much about any other form of medicine. I had seen everyone around me using natural medicines, going for massage and acupuncture, doing yoga and meditation but I had not taken much care to learn any form of healing along the way.

I started slowly. Renting a cottage in the valley we lived in and just accepting at first the few farm workers that noticed my presence as they walked past on their way to work or shop. I spent time with them, was sympathetic to their plight and did not ask more than their medical aid or pocket would allow. There was at first lots of time to study and get myself back into thinking like a doctor.

Becoming a drug-free doctor

The first major challenged happened as I was studying and getting familiar again with drugs. I knew drugs had side effects but suddenly reading about these side effect with the eyes and mind of someone who had spent years seeking out organic food, healthy medicine, eco-friendly ways of living, meditation and yoga was an eye opener that changed everything .

The average person does not realise I think that doctors don't really consider deeply that all drugs are very serious chemicals which can cause harm and even kill. It would make the practice of medicine very difficult if doctors had to keep this foremost in their minds. Instead doctors think that the benefits are worth the risk and so focus on the benefits without paying much attention to the serious toxic effects that these drugs could cause.

The realisation of the serious nature of drugs and how they could even kill was a real shock and made it increasingly difficult for me to write out a prescription for any drug apart from antibiotics. I was aware of alternatives and kept seeking ways of replacing drugs with natural therapies.

I had seen how safe they were compared to drugs and studying the side effects of drugs again reminded me why I had left medicine in the first place and that I did not want to become a conventional medical doctor prescribing drugs, which were dangerous and did not seem to be curative. Patients were generally required to take many drugs for the rest of their lives.

So the first big decision I made in returning back to the practice of medicine was to become a specialist in the non-drug treatment of disease and this decision started my journey to discover natural ways to replace drugs. My focus in these early days was based on my conventional training of disease diagnosis and then treating that disease. I continued to make a diagnosis of disease and treat the disease with natural medicine.

In those early days I knew very little about natural medicines and the great range that was available but it was clear to me that most of the farm workers I saw had an extremely poor diet and so that was a good way to start. It seemed pretty obvious that eating refined and junk food could not possibly contribute to good health and was possibly the most important cause of much of their ill health, especially for the high incidence of diabetes I was already beginning to deal with.

Using simple diets and natural remedies

Fortunately, just at this time a nursing sister who was also working part time for a Naturopath gave me a very simple diet. My focus therefore on all my early patients was quite simple: change their diet habits and use natural products to treat their disease.

I realised also that most of these farm workers were probably deficient in a range of nutrients so I added a simple vitamin mineral supplement or brewer's yeast to the management. Some of my early clients were too poor to afford much medication so that apart from changing the diet all they received was a packet of vitamin mineral pills or the brewer's yeast tablets.

Changing the diet could not have been more simple. I knew that the workers loved their potatoes, onions, pumpkin and cabbage and so I restricted them to these foods for one month and off all refined and junk foods. Just doing that was enough to shift them fairly quickly from ill health to becoming relatively healthier. Many could come off their pain medication, anti-hypertensives and reduce other symptomatic medication.

I was astonished to see 'disease' improve and even disappear with my simple approaches. For someone trained in the use of drugs to treat disease, this was a real surprise and that drugs were not always necessary made a huge impression.

Many of the early herbal medications that I became familiar with were the toxic powerful herbs, not often used by herbalists because of their toxicity but favoured by medical doctors because that fitted very nicely into the paradigm of treating the disease.

These herbs included digitalis, colchicine, belladonna, rewolfia, and less toxic symptomatic herbs such as ginger, chamomile, peppermint and many other simple household herbs. My thinking in those early days was very much driven by my conventional medical training i.e. make a diagnosis of disease and then treat the disease and the associated symptoms.

The only difference from my conventional colleagues was that I very seldom used drugs and instead just changed the diet and used mainly simple and some toxic herbs which were strong enough to improve the patient's symptoms. Many of these latter herbs are still used by the medical profession today. Colchicine is used by many doctors to treat gout. Digitalis and rewolfia are now regarded as old fashioned but in some countries are still used because they work well and are inexpensive.

The above management protocols were the first phase of my shifting focus towards becoming an Integrative Doctor i.e. shifting from using drugs to treat disease to using natural medicines to treat the disease. The second phase was more subtle and crept up on me and in a way was another eureka moment.

It suddenly occurred to me that everything I was doing was not really treating the disease but supporting health and that as health improved, the health within the body would then do the healing and the ill health would slowly resolve and even the disease symptoms would improve or even disappear. This would take time of course. The disease developed slowly as described in earlier chapters but if health could heal then it would.

Changing the diet, giving simple vitamin and mineral supplements, adding a few herbs were often enough to shift everything. At this point I knew I was onto something important. As a medical doctor I needed to pay attention to the disease but this became less interesting as I began to realise that before the disease appeared was a range of metabolic dysfunctions which were still present with the disease. These dysfunctions would increase over time until the system spiraled more and more out of control eventually ending up with 'the disease'.

In changing the diet and adding nutrients I was removing the toxic load of refined carbs and processed foods and improving the functionality of the systems within the body and as function improved, healing improved, detox improved, more energy became available and real healing was the result.

This was really unlike the approach of most other doctors who prescribe drugs. Drugs are certainly powerful enough to suppress symptoms but generally do not heal. People become dependent on the drugs and generally find it necessary to take more and more drugs over time to control their symptoms.

At last I had the feeling that I was moving in the right direction. The body's innate intelligence knew what to do and would move towards better health provided it was given the nutrients required and if the various blocks to the flow of healing discussed in previous chapters were removed.

Remove blocks, nourish and the body will heal itself

My practice started to fill up with people who were unhappy with taking drugs that did not always make them feel better, that were becoming addicting and that their disease anyway continued to progress slowly but surely. More and more medical failures came to see me. These were patients doing the rounds from one doctor to another, frustrated beyond measure that their disease remained as persistent as ever and that even the best medical specialist could do little to help apart from prescribing the next expensive drug that often still had unknown side effects.

My enthusiasm was sorely tested during these early years as I realised that this was not going to be easy. Changing the diet and adding a few supplements was not going to work for everyone. Ill health was a great deal more complex than I thought.

I needed another eureka moment to help me in this journey.

Introducing acupuncture and low energy laser into my practice

One of the techniques I learnt very early on in my practice was acupuncture. Acupuncture was probable one of the primary reasons for the success of my practice in those early days. When used for the right indications the results were often spectacular.

I soon became well known for treating chronic headaches and back pain in particular. Some of the results verged almost on the miraculous with curative results even in people who had suffered for years and had consulted with one doctor or specialist after another. I remember one lady who had not been able to lie flat in bed for some years. She slept instead in a TV recliner that could move back slightly. It was the longest set of acupuncture treatments I ever did, perhaps as many as twenty treatments, but slowly and surely her pain diminished and by the time she stopped coming, lying down was easy.

In another case I remember, a farmer came to see me with a frozen shoulder, which he had suffered from for almost one year. A single needle place in a point below his knee released the shoulder in a dramatic way. There were astonishing other cures in many other conditions as well, such as shingles, neuralgias, knee and shoulder pains and many other aches and pains around the body.

Even to this day, thirty years after using my first acupuncture needle, I am still surprised at the results of inserting a few simple acupuncture needles. A placebo response? Well maybe but the next technique I learnt made it much more difficult for me to dismiss the needle effect as 'just a placebo'.

The device that contributed to my learning curve and many very satisfied patients is called a low-energy laser. Surgeons use high-energy lasers as a surgical tool for cutting through tissue. A 50-watt laser will burn a hole through the body but when used in low power from 1 mw to even 100 mw, instead of a destructive effect there is a stimulation of healing.

There is much good research to confirm the benefits of low energy lasers. There are world conferences, journals, books and hundreds if not thousands of medical journal articles on the use of low-energy lasers. It seems that the cells of the body not only emit photons or light particles but that photons can also activate physiological processes.

My own experience confirms this healing potential of the laser. Like acupuncture, the results of the laser can be almost instantaneous with further improvement following each therapy session. The laser and acupuncture can treat similar conditions but there are areas where one may not choose to use needles, where the laser is the preferred method. This includes the breast, eye, anus, vagina, certain internal organ problems and when treating children and babies. Breast pain and anal fissures for example will generally respond to the first treatment with continued recovery following each treatment given a few days later.

My Personal Journey

The low energy laser was able to eliminate the possible role of the placebo. Firstly, the light I used cannot be seen (infra-red), secondly, there is no sensation felt and thirdly, people often thought I was merely doing some test on them and yet there were still very often dramatic effects. The look on their face after this apparent 'test' with the pain often 50% or more improved was always a great pleasure to behold.

I can truly say that my results with acupuncture and the low energy laser really made my practice up in the mountains and a good distance from the nearest town a great success and within a year or two of opening, my practice was full every day.

Some of the critical work on these low energy lasers has been performed in Russia and probably why this form of treatment is less well known in the west. This is not surprising, since western medicine has been driven by a biochemical and pharmaceutical agenda unlike that in Russia, which under the communist regime had been under the care and control of the state.

Russian researchers were intrigued by the ability of healers to lay their hands on people and initiate a healing response. This disconnect between a belief in God and healing is interesting and goes a long way in explaining the Russian interest in energy medicine and the research that began in the 1970s. Healing as in the laying of hands on the sick person by a recognised healer was not a prayer or appealing to God for help but rather an energetic transformation of energy between the healer and sick person.

Huge institutes were built in Russia financed by the state where research was begun on energy medicine starting off with simple electromagnetic fields, colour, magnetic and sound waves. Within the walls of these institutes were not only biochemists but also physicists and engineers. It was quite revolutionary to include the latter groups. Most research in the western medical model is supported by pharmaceutical companies interested in drugs and employing biochemists with very little interest in energy medicine. Energy medicine in any of its forms is generally dismissed as fringe, as alternative medicine and as unsupported by evidence based medicine.

My experience in the use of acupuncture and laser therapy opened me to another field of information that I realised was being sidelined by western medicine dominated by a biochemical and pharmaceutical paradigm. In order to investigate energy medicine further I formed the Bioenergy Association and invited a few physicists and engineers to meet once per month and discuss concepts of energy in medicine.

There was a professor of Bioengineering at the local university. 'Bio' means 'nature' and so I was very excited to discover such a position at the medical school assuming that he would be doing research on energy in living systems. Instead I discovered that all the research in that department had more to do with engineering orthopaedic hardware and other such research than anything to do with living systems and electromagnetic fields.

The meetings of the Bioenergy Association turned out to be very interesting and although my understanding of electromagnetic energy and fields was very rudimentary, I knew enough to ask tough questions and constantly brought the group to the recognition that biochemistry was clearly not enough to understand the workings of living systems.

Electromagnetism added another whole dimension to the human condition and could in theory provide answers to the riddle of ill health and how the system maintains its integrity despite emotional storms, and temperature shifts and biochemical changes from moment to moment.

The association continued to meet monthly for about two years and during this time I enlarged my understanding of what I called the greater anatomy of human beings to include energy and information.

The Greater Anatomy of human beings includes biochemistry, bioenergy and bio-information.

My journey in life had always taken two directions. My interest in medicine had always been about investigating why people got sick and how to stimulate a healing response. My other special interest is the inner journey or what is generally referred to as the spiritual journey towards discovering the higher Self as opposed to the lower self. These two aspects of my life, the outer journey as scientist trying to investigate the material world I was living in and the inner subjective world of thought, emotions, mind and consciousness has been my consuming interest.

While in the early parts of my life these two journeys seemed different and separate, they increasingly impinged on each other as my inner journey took me deeper and slowly connected the inner and outer, the subjective with the objective. As Dr Kaushik, my spiritual teacher had said, there is no difference between inner and outer, it is only my mind that makes the difference.

Connecting the inner world of spirit and outer world of matter.

Connecting the inner and outer was an important step in enlarging my worldview and changing my perspective around the cause and management of ill health. If human beings also had subjective components and these components could influence health and disease then these components had to be understood and included into the worldview of ill health.

It was for this reason that very early in my medical studies I became interested in hypnosis and the power of the mind over the body. I was fascinated by miraculous healing and people's anecdotal stories of healings that occurred through prayer. Traditional systems used their sacred rites, chanting and other symbolism to induce healing responses. My special and abiding interest however was mind and consciousness and how these faculties worked in my own experience.

The Outer Journey

My interest in healing using natural medicine has continued to this day even after retiring from active practice. I sought out natural products and techniques to heal and thought a great deal about the difference between the conventional medical model and the new Integrative model that I was involved in.

I started the South African Journal of Natural Medicine, which was sold throughout South Africa to the public and wrote monthly newsletters for Health Professionals. I started the SA Society of Integrative Medicine, which was the political arm of medical doctors wishing to practice this form of medicine.

All this time however I was seeking to simplify the approach to healing because I believed that healing was much more than just prescribing medicines, whether they were drugs or natural products, much more even than using needles or lasers, that there was a component that transcended all these modalities. I guess I was always intrigued by the magical, subjective, miraculous healings that I had read about, heard about and experienced in my own life and this vision spurred me to constantly seek further.

The Inner Journey

I had started meditation while travelling around Europe and have continued this practice on and off until today. The purpose of meditation in the early days was to attain certain 'spiritual' experiences. I somehow assumed that I could develop unconditional love, psychic abilities and inner peace by this practice. It was not that easy. My very trained western thinking mind kept getting in the way with its thoughts stirring up emotions, so that meditation was frustrating at times, while at other times it did seem to present me with interesting experiences.

Over time I was able to stop identifying with thought and merely watch the play of thought and emotions. This was a major step and while it was still 'noisy', at least the thoughts could arise and I felt somewhat detached from those thoughts. This ability to separate from the thoughts and even emotions was a major advance in my experience of meditation. I realised that thought and emotions had been my persona, who I thought I was and suddenly there were thought and emotions going on as if they had a life of their own and I was standing as 'awareness'. This awareness was clearly deeper than the thought and emotions happening in front of me.

Then one day I realised that the thoughts had stopped being an irritation and with thoughts no longer in my face all the time, emotions also calmed down and a greater sense of inner peace was a more constant presence. Thought is noisy and when emotions arise, then the noise gets even louder. If I was irritated or anxious when I sat down to meditate then it was difficult to attain this quiet inner peace.

Over time this meditative experience began filtering into my life so that it was much easier to be present as 'awareness' and merely observe the thinking mind having its own life.

Discovering inner peace and its contents beyond the thinking mind.

Dr. Kaushik, all those many years ago when I was just starting my 'spiritual' journey had said to me that the inner and outer life was really one life and not two separate lives. The truth of that statement took me forever to understand.

It was only as I discovered the depth of 'inner space' and recognised that my 'awareness' was always at the deepest level and everything else was 'in front' of awareness that I realised that the inner and outer was always merely the play of the thinking/emotional self, using thought, imagination and emotional responses to create reality. When all of the above disappeared then only awareness remained.

Reactions still happened, reminding me of the presence of ego, self-centeredness, judgment and conditioning. Clearly there is still much work to do; nevertheless finding inner peace has become easier. In particular, the recognition that thinking and all its components are always giving a limited view of reality and that therefore that part of the mind is really not in charge.

Having accepted the limitation of thinking mind in a world of extreme complexity had given me a sense of peace that had long eluded me. Thinking mind with its team of experts (imagination, emotions, conditioning) has now been identified for what it is and can do. Thinking has its place and certainly contributes enormously to the richness of my life without which I would not have got to where I am today. It is this very richness, creativeness and powerful imaging of the thinking mind that has kept me trapped within its very large sphere of control. Trying to step back from thinking using the thinking mind cannot work but using the thinking mind to recognize its own limitations has worked over time.

The problem for a long time was that the richness of thought kept me away from what seemed a rather boring 'inner peace'. This is the illusion and trap of the spiritual journey. Thinking seems so juicy compared to 'inner peace' that it is easy to talk spirituality while at the same time actually still on the side of thinking and all that comes with it i.e. judgment, reactions, points of view etc.

I am reminded of a statement in the bible around the Garden of Eden and the apple that Adam and Eve ate, despite warnings from God not to eat of these fruits. Having 'sinned by eating the fruit they were kicked out of paradise.

'You are free to eat from any tree in the garden; but you must not eat from the tree of the knowledge of good and evil, for when you eat of it you will surely die.' [1]

For a long time, perhaps years, I could choose between inner peace and still munching the apple of 'thinking'. Very slowly as I spent more

1   NIV, Genesis 2:15-17

345

time in inner peace and giving less credence to thinking I began to notice other aspects of the inner peace that I had not noticed before. This definitely made that space beyond thinking and emotions begin to feel more appealing. I noticed for example that awareness had not disappeared. I was very clearly aware of thinking and emotions so that awareness and inner peace were now clearly recognised as deeper than thinking and emotions.

I also noticed that my feeling self had not disappeared and I could clearly distinguish between emotions and feeling. I then became aware that within inner peace I could see the world differently. Instead of everything being filtered by thought, there was a purity of the world around me, a direct seeing uncluttered by interpretation and imagination.

At first thinking kept wanting to interpret everything and would keep jumping in with ideas, comparisons, comments and judgments, but as I became more comfortable with this space, thinking just stopped interfering and the purity of the view became more rich, expansive and then 'love' began to appear as a condition of this 'space'.

Everything seemed to emanate love, was soaked in love and even breathed out love. That was a surprise to me and I am having difficulty in writing about this because this love was not an emotion or even a feeling. It was more a knowing that love was presents everywhere. I could not own it or even use it because it just was, but in order to discover this love it seemed that I had to do this long journey of controlling the thinking mind and emotional reactions and stand in that place of inner peace long enough for it to reveal itself to me.

This journey has been a long one.

I now know where inner peace is. I am very clear that inner peace disappears for me when I react emotionally or allow my ego to take control again: that deep within, beyond the ego with its control over thinking and emotions there is my 'soul being' surrounded and enveloped by love and inner peace.

My journey both inner and outer continues. My three children grew up and left home, married and had their own children. I divorced my travelling companion and the mother of my children. We both realised that we had stopped growing together and needed to move on separately.

My Personal Journey

A journalist from one of the local newspapers asked for an interview. Falling in love again was really great fun even at the age of 60 years old and this started a whole new cycle of growth and going deeper. We have been together for almost 15 years. A very rich and meaningful relationship allowing a new depth of understanding, compassion and a deepening of relationship with another. This has not always been easy but it has been the measure of that relationship that the difficult times have only enriched us both rather than cause continued friction, arguments and a legacy of bad feelings.

The ability to confront difficulties, dealing with arguments and recognising that in the end each person must deal with their own reactions rather than blaming has been really good. We have worked out techniques of dealing with confrontation that brings us both back to inner peace and enlarged our compassion and love for each other and others.

The journey within is never ending. It continues to surprise in its unfolding. The secret I think is to persist in wanting to go deeper and not be distracted by the thinking mind and the barriers that the same thinking mind throws up. Letting go judgment, of self and others, not being afraid of the unknown, allowing the Great Mystery to reveal itself in each moment without covering this mystery up with mundane thinking and conditioning has been my lessons over the years.

At the age of 72 years I finally stopped my practice with patients in order to teach, write and walk my dog every morning. It has been a good life and I still look forward to each new day and the blessings it brings. Some days are difficult and some days just flow with the synchronicity of the moment. They are all blessings in disguise. They are all love expressing itself. They are all the outbreath of the Great Mystery that surround me.

To gain the pearls of the spiritual journey it seems that one must first recognize the traps of the thinking mind .

Beyond and deeper than thinking and it emotional components lies inner peace and within that peace the pearls of the journey can be discerned.

About the Author

Bernard Brom qualified as a medical doctor in 1965. While specialising in gastroenterology he became dissatisfied with medicine and his lifestyle and in 1971 gave up medicine and travelled around the world in a VW kombi for almost 6 years.

He returned to South Africa and started an integrative medical practice. He very soon specialised in the non-drug treatment of ill-health, and after studying Traditional Chinese Medicine (TCM), herbal medicine and homeopathy realised that conventional medicine's focus on disease had moved doctors away from lifestyle management and how to support health.

Instead of focusing on TCM and alternative therapies he immersed himself in exploring how a person becomes ill and how to support the person back to previous health. This did not require breaking away from the conventional medical model, but rather shifting the focus away from the disease model and the use of dangerous drugs towards lifestyle medicine and supporting health medicine. His approach was that while treating the disease and symptomatic approaches using drugs had their place, it needed to be within a model of medicine that was much more supportive to health improvement.

Dr Brom was chairman of the South African Acupuncture Medical Association and the founder and chairman of the South African Society of Integrative Medicine (SASIM). He was also one of the founders and the first Chairman of the Traditional and Natural Health Alliance, an organisation working towards a balanced and appropriate regulatory process for natural products.

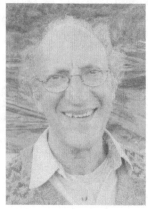

He has also written extensively on integrative medicine, both in medical journals and in his monthly newsletters. He founded the Complementary Medicine Journal in 1996 which became the Journal of Natural Medicine in 2000.

His non-medical interests include walking in nature, growing organic vegetables, deep discussion on the meaning of life and his own inner spiritual journey.

Dr Bernard Brom

Index

Index

Index

Probiotics 183

Prozac 223, 253

psychological health 180

Psycho-spiritual 56

Q

Qi 29, 89

R

Reductionism 40, 43, 46

reductionistic 47-48

Reformation 36

Rheumatoid arthritis 178

Ritalin 292

Roman Catholic Church 36

Rudolph Steiner 61

S

SAMe 182

Sagan, Carl 39

Sanchez A 181

Sarles H, 250

Segerstrom SC 151

Selenium 130, 192

Self-Healing 101

Sheldrake, Rupert 300

Singh RB 280

Sleep 199, 296

Smuts, General Jan 41, 45

Spontaneous remission 206

Steiner, Rudolph 61

Stomach Acid 203

Stress 122, 233

sugar 277

Symptomatic treatment 48

Systemic lupus erythematosis 178

T

Tarnopolsky, Dr. Mark 285

Telemetry 166

tiredness 295

Thompson, Francis 97

Thymus extract 183

Thyroid hormone deficiency 295

Tobacco 134

Toxic Environment 127, 129, 131, 133, 135, 137, 139, 141

Toxins 119

Traditional Chinese Medicine 11, 28, 65, 81, 106, 211, 214

Trousseau, Armand 244

V

vitalists 35

Vitamin A 192

Vitamin Bs 192

Vitamin C 20, 191

Vitamin D 182, 191, 286

Vitamins 19, 20

Vitamins and minerals 18

W

Walker,Labadarios et al 274

Wheaton A 125